THE HOME PHARMACY

Dr Vernon Coleman

THE HOME PHARMACY

The Consumer's Guide to
Over-the-counter Medicine

This book is not intended as a substitute for the medical advice of physicians. The reader should consult a physician in all matters relating to health and particularly in respect of any symptoms which may require diagnosis or medical attention. Whilst the advice and information are believed to be true and accurate at the time of going to press, neither the author nor the publisher can accept any legal responsibility or liability for any errors or omissions that may be made.

ISBN: 0 333 27506 3

First published 1980 by
MACMILLAN LONDON LIMITED
4 Little Essex Street London WC2R 3LF
and Basingstoke
Associated companies in Delhi Dublin Hong Kong
Johannesburg Lagos Melbourne New York Singapore
and Tokyo

In Association with Pan Books

Printed in Great Britain by
BILLING & SONS LIMITED
Guildford, London and Worcester

CONTENTS

ACKNOWLEDGEMENTS

When I started to write this book I discovered, to my horror, that there is no complete list of home medicines in existence. Not even the magnificently comprehensive *Martindale's Extra Pharmacopoeia* contains the names of all the products available over the chemist's counter without prescription.

To acquire details of the hundreds of products included in this book I wrote to several hundred private and public companies and retailers asking for help and information. Despite the fact that many of the people to whom I wrote must have had considerable misgivings about the usefulness (to them) of the book I planned to write, most were helpful and courteous. I would like to thank them and hope that I have not offended too many of them!

In addition to commercial enterprises I wrote to a number of trade and professional associations and institutions. Once more my inquiries invariably brought useful and important material. My thanks, therefore, are due to the staffs of these organizations. Also I owe thanks to the many pharmacists who so kindly gave me advice.

For helping me with copies of journals and texts, I am grateful to Mrs L. van Aernsbergen, Mrs Sheila Pallister and the rest of the staff at the Royal Society of Medicine, and to Miss E. M. Edward and Mrs N. English of the Sir John Black Library at the Warwickshire Postgraduate Medical Centre.

Special thanks go to Kyle Cathie of Pan Books who suggested that I write this book and who provided guidance and encouragement throughout its preparation, to Eileen Reynolds who translated many pages of my illegible typing, to Hetty Thistlethwaite who patiently nursed the typescript through several stages, and to those professional advisers who read the typescript and offered much valuable advice. Despite all their help final responsibility for the contents of the book is, of course, mine.

Finally, as ever, my thanks to my wife, Peggy, who helped in a thousand and one practical ways but most of all by simply being there.

Vernon Coleman, 1980

PREFACE

Most people have at some time or other gone into a chemist's shop and been confused by the wide assortment of medicines available for any specific ailment. If you want something for indigestion which of the dozens of different products should you choose? The pharmacist will probably be busy dispensing medicines and the counter assistants may have little idea of the real merits of the alternative choices.

The manufacturers' claims may be helpful and they may be misleading. But even when they're informative they don't help you to differentiate between rival claims.

If you have ever had that problem then this book is written for you. It is designed to help you decide for yourself what is the best buy. You will be able to decide whether or not the most expensive brand is the best and to choose a product that is likely to be most effective, most convenient and safest for you.

There are many thousands of products sold with the intention of preventing disease or treating illness. Simply compiling a list of the medicines available proved far more difficult than I had imagined. No such list previously existed and huge credit is due to the many people and organizations who helped me prepare this list and investigate the claims and counter-claims of several hundred manufacturers.

In two of my previous books – *The Medicine Men* and *Paper Doctors* – I castigated various sections of the medical profession for making claims which I considered to be unreasonable. Members of 'fringe' medicine groups who welcomed the criticisms I made then can hardly complain if in this book I have felt it necessary to say harsh things about some of their assertions. I think it is relevant to point out that I have no connection whatsoever with any company or organization involved in the preparation, marketing or sale of any medicine. My sole aim has been to write an honest and useful book.

I have tried to approach each product and group of products with an open mind, expecting neither to praise nor condemn until I had studied both sides of each argument and weighed the evidence. Nevertheless, I am well aware that it is physically impossible for any one person to study all the available literature relating to home medicines. In one recent twelve-month period the World Health Organization collected 40,000 reports about viral infections alone. Even super-specialists, dealing with well-defined areas of medicine, claim that they are unable to read all the relevant books and journals. In addition, it is possible that while this book is at the printer's new evidence about available treatments may be published.

In order to ensure that no reader suffers either through my ignorance or through the appearance of new information I have remained unashamedly conservative while assessing the evidence, recommending only those products which seem to me to be both safe and effective. In the end, whatever information I have collected, the opinions are my own.

This book does not contain advice on the diagnosis of illness or the nursing of sick patients and it is not intended as an alternative to medical advice. It is simply a guide to the medicines which can be properly used in the home and if there is any doubt about the correct diagnosis and treatment then medical advice should be sought. This book simply offers my personal views on the benefits and qualities of alternative remedies.

I have assumed that the people using the book will be capable of judging for themselves whether they have indigestion, constipation or worms. I have, however, made appropriate suggestions about prevention and about when to seek expert advice.

I have not included the prices of drugs in this book since prices vary from shop to shop and from month to month, but readers should be able to discern from the information I have given which product is likely to be the most suitable and economic buy for them. As a general rule products which do not carry a brand name but which are labelled with the medical name followed by the letters BP or BPC will be cheaper than nationally advertised brands containing an equivalent drug.

If at any time in the future you come across a product that does not appear in the text or which seems to differ from the product I have described I would like to hear from you. Manufacturers are constantly adding new items to their lists and amending existing formulae. I apologize in advance to any manufacturers whose products have been omitted from the lists in this book. I have tried to list every product but the omission of any medicine does not mean that it is not as effective, safe and useful as listed products, or that the manufacturer's claims are suspect. If you have any comments about specific treatments or general advice which you think would be useful to future readers of this book I would be grateful if you would write to me c/o the publishers.

INTRODUCTORY NOTE

The drugs that you can buy without a prescription may be described in several different ways. They are sometimes known as proprietary medicines – although this phrase may also occasionally be used to describe those medicines which are available only on prescription. They may, on occasion, be called 'non-ethical drugs' to distinguish them from 'ethical' products, which is another name sometimes used for drugs that are only available with a prescription from a doctor. People in the medical and pharmaceutical professions describe them as OTCs, these three letters referring to the phrase 'over-the-counter' medicines, while many members of the public use the phrase 'patent medicines' to describe anything that can be bought freely and which is advertised.

To avoid confusion I have decided to use the single phrase 'home medicines' to describe all the drugs which may be bought over the counter to prevent or treat an illness. I shall use this phrase to cover both the medicines which are manufactured and sold as individual commercial products (such as *Alka Seltzer* or *Disprin*) and the medicines (such as *Soluble Aspirin Tablets BP*) which are simply prepared according to national standards and which are not manufactured or promoted by a single company (these drugs usually have the letters BP (British Pharmacopoeia) or BPC (British Pharmaceutical Codex) after their names to denote that they have been prepared according to official regulations).

Part 1 of the book is intended to provide a short background to the use of home medicines. I have taken care to include only information which is likely to be of interest to the reader who has a purely practical interest in the selection and use of home medicines. I am afraid that the professional student, looking for detailed historical, legal or pharmacological background material, will have to look elsewhere.

I have briefly described the way in which home medicines are manufactured, advertised and sold and the laws which govern their availability since it seems to me that these are factors which must have some influence on a customer selecting a medicine. I have also described the dangers associated with the use of home medicines and, in view of growing interest in 'fringe' and 'natural' remedies, I have discussed alternative medicines. In a section entitled 'Drugs and your body' I have tried to provide some food for thought!

PART 1

THE MANUFACTURE AND MARKETING OF HOME MEDICINES

A SHORT HISTORY

Although the qualities of individual drugs had been well described by the ancient Egyptians who listed and used a total of 975 medicinal remedies, by the Greeks who had a book in which the uses of 600 plants were outlined, and by many other early physicians, it was not until the seventeenth and eighteenth centuries that drugs specially made and marketed for home use (as opposed to use by health care professionals) became prominent and popular.

Many of these products relied more on imaginative advertising than their physical properties to attract customers. As we now know, even products which are totally devoid of active ingredients may have a dramatic effect on some patients. Sugar pills, which contain nothing more mystical than ordinary sugar, can be used to treat a wide range of several conditions. The patient responds to the suggestion made by the advertiser or prescriber and gets better because he believes in the potential efficacy of the product he's taking rather than because of any inherent qualities of the drug.

So, such scientifically unproven products as the *Carbolic Smoke Ball, Daffy's Elixir, Dr Bateman's Pectoral Drops, Dr Scott's Electric Hairbrush, Dr Swayne's Consumption Cure, Goddards Drops, James Morison's Universal Vegetable Compound, Samuel Lee's Bilious Pills,* and *Widow Read's Ointment for the Itch* made large sums of money for their manufacturers and distributors and undoubtedly relieved many inconvenient symptoms.

BIG BUSINESS

The manufacture and sale of home medicines today is big business.

This may seem a very obvious thing to say but it is an important point to make clear because many of the people who go into a chemist's shop or who read manufacturers' advertisements undoubtedly regard everyone associated in any way with medical care as being fired by the purest of motives.

Unfortunately, this is not quite the case. A little healthy scepticism is called for when claims and advertisements are being considered.

The truth is that the preparation and sale of home medicines in Britain alone is worth considerably more than £200 million a year. That means that on average each household spends 21p a week on medicines and that despite the National Health Service home medicines attract many buyers. There are several thousand different products on the market and in the areas where the greatest sales can be made – cold remedies, painkillers, laxatives, antacids and skin treatments – there is considerable competition.

All this means that home medicines are marketed in exactly the same way as soap powders, baked beans and aftershave lotions are marketed. Potential purchasers need to remember that.

The evidence supporting the safety and effectiveness of most home medicines has never been subjected to critical review. When over-the-counter medicines in America were recently subjected to scientific evaluation it was found that over three-quarters of the drugs studied were less effective than their manufacturers had claimed.

GIVING THE PEOPLE WHAT THEY WANT

It is far better commercially to provide people with what they want than with what is good for them. And that is why so many ineffective medicines are manufactured and sold. There are a number of popular fallacies relating to home medicines that encourage manufacturers to prepare medicines that offer little in the way of relief but a good deal in the way of promise.

Patients popularly prefer medicines that contain many ingredients. And so there are a large number of medicines that contain very small quantities of many ingredients. As a basic principle it is hardly ever worthwhile buying a home medicine that contains more than three or four active ingredients. The chances are that each ingredient will be included in such a minute quantity that it can never do any good at all. Putting ten or a dozen ingredients into one bottle of medicine is about as logical as putting ten or a dozen sauces and spices into a single bottle. The resulting sorry mixture is unlikely to be good for anything.

Another popular myth is that if a medicine is new it will be good. A nineteenth-century physician called Sir William Gull was so annoyed by the claims made by manufacturers of treatments for rheumatic fever that he published a tongue-in-cheek paper extolling the virtues of mint as a cure. The joke backfired because his mint water treatment became fashionable simply because it was new.

A third way to please potential buyers is to offer them a product that seems unusual and rather mysterious. Garlic and ginseng, for example, which do have some medicinal effects, have achieved a great deal of popularity, but no one really knows much about them apart from the fact that they have been used in strange, out-of-the-way places for centuries.

Many preparations which are offered are intended to satisfy the purchaser's vanity as much as anything else. Pharmacies are well stocked with muscle building, skin freshening, breast boosting, hair restoring products. Slimming medicines and devices are more popular than ever these days.

Finally, it is a fact that many manufacturers take advantage of the fears of patients. In recent years various cancer cures have been offered which, in my opinion, are nothing but rubbish. These treatments build false hopes and endanger those who take them. The people who make these products should be condemned to consume them interminably. People who are ill are particularly gullible and susceptible to the claims of dishonest advertisers. It is a sad but true fact that if you fill a bottle with coloured water and call it the Elixir of Life people will buy it by the gallon.

CONTROLS ON ADVERTISING

There was a time when manufacturers of home medicines could make whatever claims they liked for their products. Consequently the businessman with a greater regard for money than for truth could promote medicines as offering a cure for cancer, tuberculosis, venereal disease or any other serious disorder. Some products were, indeed, advertised as cures for *all* these conditions. Many members of the public undoubtedly believed this.

Today it is no longer possible for a manufacturer to make outrageously dishonest claims about suggested cures for serious diseases. There are official regulations which prohibit the promotion of a product for use at home if it is not suitable for use in that way. It is now illegal to promote directly to the public medicines that are available only on prescription. And medicines must sometimes be accompanied by warnings if there is sufficient doubt about their usefulness or safety. If anyone falsely describes a medicinal product he is theoretically liable to imprisonment and a large fine.

Given the extent of the existing legislation it is perhaps surprising that so many misleading advertisements do appear. There are several reasons for this. Firstly, the regulations which govern the advertising of herbal, homoeopathic and other non-traditional medicines are less stringent than the regulations which govern the promotion of traditional medicines. And secondly, because there are about 24,000 medicinal products on the market of which a large number have not yet been properly assessed, either for efficacy or for safety, the regulations are rather hollow in practical terms.

Apart from official regulations there are some voluntary rules which supposedly help to ensure that members of the public are not exposed to inaccurate advertising of home medicines.

Companies which are members of the European Associations of Manufacturers of Home Medicines are required to observe an advertising code which includes the following statements:

1 Advertisements must not be either intentionally or unintentionally misleading, or open to misinterpretation.
2 Advertisements must never promise relief or a cure.
3 An advertisement should be clearly distinguishable by the ordinary reader from the editorial content of the medium in which it appears.

Each of these suggestions has been broken by British manufacturers.

The Proprietary Association of Great Britain, an organization which represents a large number of major British home medicine manufacturers, has also published a Code of Standards of Advertising Practice which, if it were followed, would prevent any dishonest or misleading advertising matter ever reaching newspapers, magazines, radio or television. Unfortunately many of the principles in the Code are regularly ignored by British manufacturers.

Many organizations (including the Proprietary Association of Great Britain, the Advertising Association, the Newspaper Publishers Association, the Incorporated Society of British Advertisers and the Institute of Practitioners in Advertising) support the British Code of Advertising Practice which contains several pages of notes about the proper way to advertise home medicines. If you read the Code and at the same time study a collection of British magazines and newspapers the only possible conclusion that you can come to is that many of the advertisements which appear in British magazines and newspapers are written and authorized by people who do not belong to any of these august-sounding bodies.

It is, for example, forbidden to advertise bust developers, arthritis treatments and hair restoratives, and the advertising of vitamins and minerals should, it is suggested, be limited.

The Code of Advertising Practice is full of good intentions but for all practical purposes it is as relevant to the advertising and sale of home medicines as are the Laws of Cricket.

THE TOP TEN HOME MEDICINE CATEGORIES

Painkillers are probably the best-selling category of home medicine. During one recent year there were no less than four painkilling products on which manufacturers spent over half a million pounds sterling on advertisements. On one product, *Anadin*, over a million pounds was spent. Half that amount was spent on each of *Aspro Clear, Disprin* and *Phensic*, while slightly less was spent on *Hedex*.

Indigestion remedies are only slightly less enthusiastically advertised. The advertising bill for three leading products, *Alka Seltzer, Rennies* and *Setlers* came to over a million pounds in one year. And four top cold remedies – *Beechams Powders, Lem-Sip, Night Nurse* and *Vicks MediNite* – had approximately two million pounds spent on them in a single year!

The top ten categories of home medicines are as follows:

1 Cough and cold remedies
2 Painkillers
3 Vitamins

4 Indigestion remedies
5 Germicides and antiseptics
6 Laxatives
7 Tonics
8 Rubs and liniments
9 Eye preparations
10 Foot care products

Slimming preparations and baby care products would probably figure prominently on this list if it were possible to assess accurately the amount of money spent on the purely medicinal products in those categories.

CHEMISTS AND PHARMACISTS

THE ROLE OF THE PHARMACIST

Not all chemists' shops have a qualified pharmacist (the proper name for a chemist) on the premises. The ones that do not have a pharmacist are not allowed to sell drugs that have to be prescribed by a doctor, nor can they sell medicines that are not on the General Sale List.

Shops with a pharmacist in attendance are sometimes described as 'dispensing chemists' or simply 'pharmacies'. The resident pharmacist (who may own the shop or work for the owner) will be a member of the Pharmaceutical Society and entitled to have the letters MPS after his name.

During their training pharmacists have to study the ways in which medicines are prepared and how they work, and they are also taught about the side effects of drugs and the dangers of mixing medicines. Many pharmacists claim that they know more about drugs than doctors do and some of them are probably right. They are not, however, taught about the diagnosis or treatment of illness and so they are better able to offer advice about minor illnesses than major ones.

WHEN TO GO TO A PHARMACIST

It is estimated that in an average sort of year the average sort of person has one cold, one attack of muscle strain, one bout of indigestion and one burst of diarrhoea.

Naturally, there is no such creature as the 'average person' but these are the sort of problems that a pharmacist can help with. Each general practitioner in Britain has an average of 2500 patients to look after and if each one of these visited the surgery for these minor problems the GP would see thirty of these minor problems *every day*. He would have even less time to spend with the more seriously ill.

HOW TO GET THE BEST OUT OF THE PHARMACIST

If you aren't sure what medicine to buy and you want help then decide before you go into the shop exactly what you want advice about. Make sure that you see the pharmacist and not an assistant who may have been working in the shop for no more than a few days and who may know less than you do about home medicines. If the pharmacist recommends a branded product you may be able to buy an alternative BP or BPC preparation which will probably be cheaper and just as effective. Ask him.

Make sure before you leave the shop that you know when to take the medicine and how much to take. The instructions should be on the bottle or container. Ask him how long the medicine will keep and whether there are any special storage instructions. And remember that if your symptoms persist or get worse you need to see a doctor. Obey the five-day rule: if you aren't better or improving in five days – see a doctor.

THE PHARMACIST AND FIRST AID

The Chemists Defence Association recently reviewed the first aid procedures that would be regarded as normal business for a retail pharmacist. They came to the conclusion that a qualified chemist could be expected to: give advice on the treatment of minor ailments such as coughs, colds, intestinal upsets, verrucas, warts and minor foot problems; provide simple first aid assistance by removing splinters, treating minor cuts and bruises, and taking grit from a customer's eye.

They also decided that it would *not* be reasonable to expect a pharmacist to remove foreign bodies from ears or noses; to syringe ears; or to provide or suggest treatment for more serious disorders.

It is only reasonable to point out that pharmacists do not get paid to provide first aid services and therefore even the most conscientious Samaritan might feel resentful if he were continually asked for help from customers who bought all their home medicine at the local supermarket.

THE LAW AND HOME MEDICINES

There are a number of laws governing the sale of drugs. Although this is not the right place to begin a comprehensive survey of the existing legislation it will perhaps be useful if I explain something about the ways in which different drugs are controlled.

The simplest dividing line is the one which separates the drugs which can be purchased freely without a doctor's prescription and the drugs which can only be obtained with a prescription. Naturally, any drug in the first category must inevitably also be in the second category. In other words, doctors can prescribe all the drugs which can be bought freely over the counter in addition to the drugs that cannot be bought freely. Aspirin, for example, is often prescribed by doctors as a mild painkiller and an anti-inflammatory drug but it is readily available without a prescription and I doubt if there are many homes in the country in which there is not a bottle of aspirin tablets.

Sometimes the very same *brands* of medicines that are prescribed can be bought. For example, many of the drugs which are taken to alleviate indigestion, gastritis and other stomach troubles are available both with and without a prescription. You can buy *Aludrox* and *Asilone* quite freely and these are the very brands of antacid commonly prescribed by family doctors.

The group of drugs that can only be obtained *with* a doctor's prescription includes powerful painkillers, drugs for the treatment of cancer, tranquillizers and antibiotics. This group is further divided. The most powerful and potentially most dangerous drugs are subject to the most stringent controls and have to be prescribed and dispensed with particular care.

The group of drugs that can be obtained *without* a prescription, the drugs with which this book is concerned, are also divided into different categories. Some are available only from a chemist's shop where a qualified chemist is in attendance; some are available from general stores and supermarkets; and a third group, available in limited quantities only, are available from automatic machines. Naturally, all the drugs in the third group are included in the second category and all the drugs in both these categories are included in the first category. So the range of drugs available from a chemist's shop is fairly wide whereas the range of drugs available from a supermarket or public house dispensing machine is severely limited.

The laws which control the groups into which drugs are placed are complex and ever changing. Inevitably this means that it has not been practicable to describe precisely the legal categories of all the drugs described in this book. However, all the products mentioned *are* available without a prescription at the present time and are likely to remain widely available. They can, furthermore, be obtained from any qualified pharmacist or from a chemist's shop where a pharmacist is in attendance. And I do recommend that except in an emergency all home medicines are purchased from such a shop.

Finally, if you are regularly taking a medicine prescribed by a doctor and your supply runs out while you are away from home, or when your doctor is not available, you may be able to obtain a small supply from a pharmacist to last for three days (or for five days if the three days includes a public holiday) as long as your drug is not on a 'controlled' list and you can persuade the pharmacist that your need is genuine.

ALTERNATIVE MEDICINES IN THE HOME

Dissatisfaction with allopathic or traditional medicine has enlarged the opportunities for entrepreneurs offering 'fringe' medicines. Indeed, the growth in these alternative products is probably due as much to dissatisfaction with the safety and efficacy of traditional home and prescription medicines as to satisfaction experienced with the alternatives. The irony is that although traditional treatments may have been tried and found lacking in many respects, the majority of alternatives have never even been tried! Anecdotal experiences, advertising material and uncritical enthusiasm are frequently mixed up, offered and mistaken for realistic scientific judgements.

Many of the remedies which are today on the market as viable alternatives are remedies which were in regular use several hundred years ago and which are pharmacologically identical in purpose to the modern preparations which replaced them. The difference being that the modern replacements are more reliable, purer and safer. The advocates of 'natural' medicine could sometimes just as well be offering surgery without antisepsis or anaesthesia. It is probably no coincidence that some purveyors of natural medicines also sell magical cures for baldness, impotence and obesity while a few also offer for sale knickknacks, ornaments, kitchen gadgets and other ephemera.

Three of the most popular areas explored and exploited by manufacturers and retailers of alternative home medicines are biochemistry, herbalism and homoeopathy. In the following pages I have taken a closer look at these disciplines.

BIOCHEMISTRY
In addition to being a definition of the study of the chemistry of living matter the world 'biochemistry' is used to describe the philosophies put forward by a certain Dr W. R. Schuessler during the last century. Biochemistry is not a branch of homoeopathy or indeed of any speciality

– it is a discipline in its own right. Its exponents disapprove of the use of drugs and instead propose the use of inorganic, mineral substances known as 'tissue salts'.

These mineral elements, present in minute quantities in the human body, are, they insist, active and life-giving. Without them bodily rhythms are disturbed, rebuilding processes are halted and 'disease' results. A shortage or deficiency of one or more of these vital substances may result from injury, poisoning or, as one textbook on biochemistry puts it, 'obscure influences which in many instances science has not yet been able to explain'.

There are only twelve remedies used in this form of treatment: calcium fluoride, calcium phosphate, calcium sulphate, phosphate of iron, potassium chloride, potassium phosphate, potassium sulphate, magnesium phosphate, sodium chloride, sodium phosphate, sodium sulphate and silicic oxide. These are sold either individually or in various combinations. *Elasto Tablets*, sold for aching legs and advertised widely, contain calcium fluoride, calcium phosphate, phosphate of iron and magnesium phosphate.

According to the *Biochemic Handbook*, published by New Era Laboratories, who advertise and sell these twelve remedies: 'The biochemic system of medicine rests upon a firm foundation; it has stood the test of searching investigation. The more recent discoveries in the field of biological research, and the findings of present day biochemists, confirm its teachings.'

I wrote to New Era Laboratories and asked for details of these investigations. The managing director was kind enough to write back and tell me that one of their products was about to be subjected to scientific evaluation. However, until all products in the *Biochemic Handbook* have been thoroughly tested I can see no reason at all to believe that the twelve tissue salts are likely to have any useful medicinal effect on the human body. This philosophy is not so much a branch of scientific medicine as a branch of faith healing.

HERBAL REMEDIES

An advertisement for one of the largest suppliers of herbal remedies contains the following statement: 'Potter's herbal products contain no drugs whatsoever.'

Since the Shorter Oxford English Dictionary defines a 'drug' as 'an original, simple, medicinal substance, organic or inorganic, used by itself, or as an ingredient in Medicine' it is difficult to see the purpose in buying a remedy from this company!

The truth is, of course, that Potter's have been misled by the growing apprehension about drugs (sometimes thought of as being inevitably powerful, dangerous and potentially evil) into wrongly describing their own products. Any herbal remedy which has an effect on the human body is, by definition, a drug, while a product which does not have any effect on or in the body is hardly worth buying for its medicinal properties!

I think that this apparently semantic argument is an important one. Today's pharmaceutical industry uses herbal extracts as the basic ingredients for many of its despised products. Indeed, the substances sold by today's suppliers of herbal remedies appear in the major pharmaceutical textbooks. Even the common dandelion root (also known as piss-en-lit for the excellent reason that it has an effect as a diuretic) is described in *Martindale's Extra Pharmacopoeia*.

But the claims made for herbal products sometimes seem to exceed the possible scientific expectations, perhaps because many products have not yet been clinically evaluated.

One company which has done a great deal of research into the effectiveness of herbal remedies is Bio-Strath. Recognizing that herbal remedies can produce dangerous side effects and that without properly organized clinical trials claims can easily be dismissed, Bio-Strath have begun a professionally organized research programme. Their early results seem most encouraging although there is a long way to go yet before any herbal remedies can be described as definitely more effective and safer than competing pharmaceutical products.

HOMOEOPATHY

The homoeopathic science was developed by a German, Dr Samuel Christian Hahnemann, in the eighteenth century. His original theory was that the patient, who consisted of three parts – body, mind and spirit – must be treated as a whole. Disease, said Hahnemann, is a state of disorder within the patient and any treatment must be designed to restore peace and harmony, encouraging the body to protect itself rather than attempting to simply eradicate any intruding organism.

As a result, homoeopathy works on a 'hair of the dog' theory. Minute doses of drugs are given with the intention of triggering a defensive reaction within the body and stimulating the body's own natural resistance to disease, much in the same way that vaccination works.

When you are given a vaccination against smallpox a very much diluted dose of the infecting organism is injected into your body. On the basis of this sneak preview your body prepares its defences. When you are later exposed to a genuine case of smallpox and stand in danger of contracting the disease, your body has its defences ready.

The homoeopathic doctor follows what is basically a similar principle but he uses this system actually to treat existing disease rather than to prevent the development of disease.

He prescribes drugs which in larger doses will produce the very symptoms of which his patient is complaining. So, for example, he will give a vomiting patient a minute dose of ipecacuanha because that drug causes vomiting in larger quantities. And he'll give a very nervous, edgy patient a minute dose of coffee because in larger doses (such as the amount in a drink of the same name) coffee causes a greater sense of nervous awareness.

Homoeopathic doctors use a wide range of products in their attempt to trigger off this body response. They even use one drug manufactured from the black widow spider. When this spider bites a human being the symptoms are like a mild heart attack – an attack of angina. So to treat angina, homoeopathic doctors use the black widow spider. It sounds terrifying but there is a good deal of evidence that it works – not only with humans who might be influenced by the personality of the practitioners but with animals and children who are less likely to be so influenced.

The homoeopaths claim that their treatment causes very few side effects because the drugs they use are so diluted. And their claim that it is the patient they are treating and not the disease certainly sounds attractive. Certainly since the dilutions they use are enormous – they effectively empty a bottle of neat medicine into a lake and then use the lake water to treat their patients – bad reactions should be very few and very mild.

The vital point about homoeopathy is that the treatment has to be *individual*. The doctor's task is to find a drug that can produce symptoms similar to those from which the sick person is suffering and to then offer that drug in a sufficiently diluted dose. The treatment for one patient with a cold may not be the same as the treatment for another with a cold. A patient with rheumatic pains which are relieved by movement will not receive the same treatment as a patient who has rheumatic pains which are made worse by movement. In addition, the prescriber will want to know the constitutional type of the patient – both emotionally and physically.

Once all these symptoms have been identified the treatment can be arranged. Homoeopathic remedies have to be stored extremely carefully and used one at a time. The use of all other medicines has to be avoided and pollutants such as tobacco, food, drink, sweets and toothpaste must be eschewed immediately prior to taking the treatment.

It should be clear by now that homoeopathy is not a discipline to be approached lightly by amateurs. I suspect that the founder Samuel Hahnemann would have had a fit if he had seen what is being offered for sale today in the name of homoeopathy. One of the leading homoeopathic chemists pointed out to me that the word 'homoeopathic' is appropriated for various concoctions based on natural products without any regard to the real meaning of the description.

If homoeopathy attracts you then I suggest that you study an introductory guide (such as *Homoeopathy* by A. C. Gordon Ross) or contact the British Homoeopathic Association for details of the discipline and the names of homoeopathic hospitals and practitioners.

CONCLUSIONS

If you obeyed all the advertisements paid for by companies selling 'fringe' medicine products your diet would be composed of little else but garlic, ginseng, seaweed, brewer's yeast and vitamin tablets. Not the sort of diet to encourage the life insurance companies to lower your premiums, I'm afraid.

The advertisements promoting these products raise a number of strange questions. For example, how do you know if your blood needs regenerating? They also suggest that the copywriters know very little about anatomy or physiology. One advertisement I have seen describes sciatica as a type of nervousness! In fact, of course, sciatica is the name given to the type of pain which occurs when the sciatic nerve is irritated. Confusing nerve pain with nervousness is an error which does not give one much confidence in the supposedly responsible manufacturer's product.

More important, perhaps, is the fact that many of the companies selling 'natural cures', 'herbal remedies' and so on contravene many of the basic principles espoused by the innovators of the philosophies concerned.

For example, in 1747 John Wesley, an advocate of natural treatments, pointed out that it was wrong to make up compounds of twenty ingredients as apothecaries of the day were wont to do. He argued that a single, natural remedy was often more reliable. Today, of course, his successors often promote compounds containing twenty or even more natural remedies.

It is an unfortunate fact that a great many of the claims made for alternative medicines are unsubstantiated. I have looked hard for evidence supporting the various claims and have invited manufacturers and others to offer me proof that the remedies work. Little proof has been forthcoming and it is difficult to escape the conclusion that many of those selling alternative remedies are no more than charlatans taking advantage of the susceptibility and gullibility of the sick. Those who are honestly promoting their products need to work at least as hard as the pharmaceutical companies to prove the effectiveness of their products.

Where appropriate 'alternative' treatments are available they are discussed within the relevant sections of this book. But most treatments do not appear. In most cases your guess is as good as mine (or the manufacturers') as to whether the missing products are genuinely effective and until evidence is available it seems pointless to try and assess them.

DRUGS AND YOUR BODY

WHAT IS A DRUG?

Some drugs are easy to identify as such. Everyone knows that heroin is a drug and that penicillin is a drug. But what about aspirin? What about sodium bicarbonate? And what about alcohol? Is there any difference between an ordinary medicine and a drug?

According to the World Health Organization, a drug is 'any substance or mixture of substances that is manufactured, sold, offered for sale or represented for use in:

1 the treatment, mitigation, prevention, or diagnosis of disease, an abnormal physical state or the symptoms thereof in man or animal; or
2 the restoration, correction, or modification of organic function in man or animal.'

If you read that definition carefully you'll see that it includes a good many substances – some of which you may not have thought of as drugs. Aspirin, paracetamol, sodium bicarbonate, alcohol, tea and coffee are all drugs. And those 'food products' such as garlic, yeast and so on which are sold to help preserve or restore good health have to be classified as drugs, too.

PLACEBOS AND THE PLACEBO EFFECT

For decades now it has been known that approximately one-third of all patients will obtain relief from tablets and medicines which contain absolutely no pharmacologically active constituents and which work by intent rather than by physiological effect. Knowingly or unknowingly placebos are used more frequently than any other drugs.

Even patients suffering from severe pain can benefit from the placebo effect. Dozens of studies have shown that patients with severe heart pain, usually requiring major pain-relieving drugs, can obtain great relief from nothing more than sugar tablets.

It is this placebo effect which explains the effectiveness of so many home medicines – a large number of which contain nothing of any pharmacological value. For a placebo to work well the patient taking it must be convinced of the potential benefit of the product and there is no reason to suppose that advertising material is any less convincing than words of encouragement from a doctor.

Doctors still do not know exactly why or how placebos work, although recently research work has shown that when a placebo is taken special hormones are released within the brain. These hormones may then have an effect upon the body. Whatever the mechanism is we do know that a placebo will not work unless the patient taking it is convinced that he will benefit. Strong-willed, self-sufficient, suspicious folk are far less likely to benefit from the placebo effect than nervous, anxious, dependent people.

However it works the placebo effect is important and it explains the effectiveness of a large number of home medicines.

HOW DO DRUGS WORK?

Drugs can work in any one of several different ways. There are drugs which work by killing off minute organisms and thereby preventing or curing infections. There are drugs which alter the way the body works; drugs which consist of hormones or which affect the blood's clotting mechanisms fall into this group. Then there are the drugs which can actually prevent the development of disease. Vaccines, which give the human body an advance look at potential infections and therefore enable it to prepare defence mechanisms, are obviously members of this important group.

But most of the drugs that can be bought over the counter in a chemist's shop or supermarket do not cure diseases, they simply relieve symptoms. Painkilling drugs don't usually cure the disease that is producing pain (although under some circumstances they may help speed a cure) – they simply relieve the pain. Antacid drugs don't cure stomach ulcers – but they relieve the associated pains.

It is, incidentally, worth remembering that many of the symptoms home medicines are designed to eradicate are, in fact, manifestations of the body's attempt to cure itself.

Should you swallow threatening bacteria then you will begin vomiting and develop diarrhoea as your body tries to get rid of the unwanted invaders. If you do heavy work regularly then your skin will become thicker and rougher so that it is more capable of coping – you will get callouses.

Contract an infection and your body temperature will rise to try and kill off the causative organisms. Minor skin infections are sealed off as boils, and your tonsils act as barriers preventing bacteria from getting into your body.

When you have something in your eye the tears will flow in an attempt to wash the foreign body away, and when you have something caught in your throat you will automatically cough in an attempt to dislodge it.

Pain is a warning sign that should be taken seriously. If you ignore muscle pains, for example, then you are likely to do further damage. If you ignore indigestion pains for too long then you may develop a peptic ulcer.

Unhappily, we rarely appreciate the efforts that our bodies make on our behalf. Indeed most of the defence mechanisms which operate automatically are treated as unwanted. When we have an attack of diarrhoea induced by bacteria we take medicine to stop it. When we develop boils we smear them with creams which send the bacteria running for cover instead of breaking out into the open where they can easily be removed. When we're hot with an infection (as our bodies try to kill off bacteria which don't like high temperatures) we take aspirins to help cool ourselves down.

When we sweat we use powders and deodorants. When we develop callouses we soften them. When we cough we take medicines to try and stop ourselves coughing.

The very fact that home medicines work symptomatically, dealing with symptoms rather than diseases, means that they must often directly oppose these automatic defence mechanisms. Naturally it would be unrealistic to expect patients to do nothing about symptoms which are inconvenient or uncomfortable. But it is well worth remembering that your body does know best and that annoying symptoms may be early warning signs of developing disease and your body's way of protecting you.

THE DANGERS OF HOME MEDICINES

Home medicines seem bound to play an increasingly important part in everyday medical care. Medical services everywhere are under tremendous pressure with health care professionals often unable to provide more than a rudimentary service for the majority of patients and generally unwilling to provide advice for minor, self-limiting problems. In addition, the faith of patients in the available medical services has taken a heavy battering in recent years. It is sometimes said, for example, that if a patient in hospital has two diseases the chances are that the second disease was caused by the treatment for the first. Inevitably this sort of knowledge has damaged the doctor-patient relationship with the result that many people are actively interested in acquiring a rudimentary knowledge of self-help techniques.

There is, however, a warning which needs to be sounded loud and very clear. Just as doctors are likely to make mistakes when prescribing drugs, partly because of the variety and complexity of modern medicines, so patients are likely to make mistakes in self-diagnosis. And then home medicines can be just as dangerous as prescription medicines. In this section I have outlined some of the ways in which home medicines can prove to be a problem in the hope that once the risk areas are identified the dangers can be minimized.

MISLEADING SOLACE

One of the greatest hazards of home medicines is that they may lull the patient into a false sense of security by providing him with symptomatic relief or even, on occasion, by making him *feel* that they have provided him with symptomatic relief.

For example, a car industry executive noticed that about half an hour after his breakfast and half an hour before his evening meal he was getting pains across the top part of his abdomen. He decided that the pains were caused by indigestion and so he bought a bottle of antacid mixture from a local chemist's shop. It didn't help much but he thought he would persevere and so he tried a different brand.

Once or twice the pain was so bad that it actually seemed to make him breathless but the executive noticed that if he stopped and took a good swallow from his bottle of white indigestion medicine and then waited for a couple of minutes the pain and the breathlessness would both disappear.

He went on like this for six months. And then had a heart attack.

What he had been suffering from had not been indigestion but angina – an early warning sign of heart disease. The pains had developed after breakfast and before his evening meal because he walked to his office every morning and walked home again after work. The pains were brought on by exercise not hunger or food. And it was not the indigestion medicine but the rest which brought him relief.

That man's mistake could have been fatal. If he had visited a doctor after the pains had persisted instead of simply buying bottle after bottle of medicine an earlier diagnosis could have been made and that heart attack perhaps avoided.

Similarly, a patient who takes repeated doses of an antacid for what he thinks is indigestion and who actually does obtain genuine relief may well be masking the early signs of peptic ulceration. The antacid will not cure the condition and may, by delaying the time at which professional help is sought, mean that the future prognosis is not as good as it might have been.

The moral is that home medicines should be used as short-term palliatives and never as long-term solutions.

DANGEROUS INTERACTION

Many diabetic patients understand their disease extremely well, knowing a great deal about the potential complications and the hazards of disobeying instructions relating to the use of tablets, insulin or food. The shop assistant I'm about to describe was no exception.

She always watched her diet carefully and regulated her intake of sugar wisely. She took tablets every morning to help stimulate the production of insulin within her body. I was extremely surprised when she went out of control and had to be taken into hospital unconscious.

Her problem had simply been that in an attempt to cure a persistent cough she had swallowed bottlefuls of a well-known brand of cough medicine. The cough medicine contained a large quantity of sugar and had been quite enough to throw her diabetes out of control.

The moral here is that anyone who suffers from a chronic, long-term disease or who takes medicines prescribed by a doctor should not take any home medicine without their doctor's permission. Combinations between some prescribed and non-prescribed medicines can be fatal.

THE HAZARDS OF THE MEDICATION ITSELF

Home medicines can easily cause major side effects when they are used improperly. Used at the proper dose for the proper length of time they are relatively safe. Used at the wrong dose for too long they can be just as fatal as much more powerful drugs.

One patient I remember very well had been taking aspirin tablets every day for many years. She didn't know that she was taking aspirin tablets because she was taking a well-known branded product that is frequently advertised on the television as an effective painkiller. She took these pills daily because she believed that they helped to prevent monthly period pain. The absence of period pain seemed to simply confirm her belief in the efficacy of her home treatment. Just as the man who claims that elephant powder keeps elephants away can prove it by pointing to the absence of elephants in the neighbourhood.

I saw her when she first started to complain of stomach pains. She had given herself gastritis which cleared up quickly and completely once she had abandoned her silly and damaging habit.

A comprehensive survey of the hazards associated with home medicines would fill several thousand pages. Even apparently 'safe' substances like vitamins can be dangerous if the recommended dose is exceeded. Throughout this book I have tried to describe some of the commoner hazards associated with the commoner home medicines. **To avoid mistakes and side effects always read carefully the manufacturer's recommendations and warnings.**

Many of the products listed in this book carry manufacturers' recommendations and warnings which should never be ignored.

Warnings obviously vary according to the constituents of particular products but there are four major ones which recur quite frequently. These are:

1   Do not exceed the stated dose.
2   Keep out of the reach of children.
3   Do not take if you are already on medicines prescribed by a doctor.
4   Do not continue with treatment if symptoms persist.

These warnings are worth adopting as general rules. In my opinion symptoms should be considered persistent if they last for more than five days. (Obviously *some* symptoms need medical advice well before five days!)

OVERDOSES

Any medicine that can do good can also do harm and, taken in excess, may prove fatal. Even ordinary iron tablets, taken to protect a patient from developing anaemia or to correct an existing case of anaemia, may kill if taken in too large a quantity by too small a child.

Domestic accidents are an important cause of death nowadays and accidental and deliberate self-poisoning with drugs are two of the major types of domestic accidents. In all it is estimated that no less than one in ten of all medical admissions to hospital are adults who have been poisoned by drugs. An adult in Britain today is more likely to die as a result of poisoning by some chemical substance than he or she is to die in any of the violent ways most of us fear. In the last year for which statistics are available a total of 3977 people died of chemical poisoning while the fatal victims of plane crashes, train crashes, fires, drowning accidents, industrial accidents and homicides added up to 2685.

Many other accidental poisonings involve children and it is vital to remember to keep all medicines locked up and well out of reach. There are some 40,000 poisoning or suspected poisoning cases involving children under fifteen in England and Wales every year, and in some large cities more children die from pill poisoning than from measles, german measles, poliomyelitis, tuberculosis, rheumatic fever, scarlet fever and streptococcal infections put together.

To avoid these dangers it is important not only to keep medicines safely (in childproof bottles) but to throw away all old medicines. Keep only what you're really likely to use or need. And if you suspect anyone of having taken an overdose, whether by design or accident, seek expert advice at once and show the expert the bottle from which the overdose was most likely to have been taken. Symptoms of accidental poisoning include vomiting, unconsciousness, drowsiness and sweating.

MEDICINES AND ALCOHOL

Inside the body medicines and alcohol are often broken down into their constituent parts in similar ways, using the same organs. They may also have similar side effects. Naturally this means that if you're taking a medicine and you also drink alcohol the effects of both may be heightened and prolonged. Neither the drug nor the alcohol can be broken down and metabolized at the normal speed. Antihistamines, cold cures and cough medicines are particularly likely to be a problem.

So if you're taking medicines don't drink. Since home medicines should only be used for a few days at a time the deprivation will not be too dreadful.

DRIVING UNDER THE INFLUENCE

If there are six vehicles waiting in a queue the chances are high that at least one driver will be under the influence of drugs. I don't mean heroin, hashish or cocaine but medicines legally prescribed by a doctor or bought from a pharmacist.

A large variety of different drugs may affect your ability to drive (or operate a fork lift truck, combine harvester or motor bike or navigate a boat or climb a church steeple). Naturally many of the drugs which affect the driver's ability are prescribed products. Drugs given for anxiety or depression and powerful painkillers can be a problem. But there are also many products which are obtainable without a prescription which can cause difficulties.

Drugs taken for hay fever and allergies in general are particularly likely to cause drowsiness. Every year a manufacturer comes out with a new product that is said not to cause drowsiness. So far most of these claims should be treated with reservation. Travel sickness pills can cause drowsiness too. My wife and I once took some tablets to stop sea sickness when crossing the Channel and though we weren't sick we didn't wake up properly until we had been in Paris for two days.

Medicines for coughs and colds need to be taken with care too – they often contain antihistamines.

Always ask the chemist if it is safe to drive while taking a particular product. Or at least read the product label and leaflet. Don't mix drugs, or drugs and alcohol, and do follow instructions carefully. It's often a good idea to try out a drug you haven't used before some time when you are not going to be driving. If you do not drive at the weekend then try it out then. Alternatively use public transport while you experiment with the product.

ADDICTION

People can and do get addicted to the strangest things. There was recently a report in the *British Medical Journal* of a woman who became addicted to *Dettol*. More commonly people have become addicted to cough medicines and anti-diarrhoeal medicines.

There are, of course, different types of addiction. Some people become physically addicted on particular drugs, others become psychologically dependent, and yet more simply develop bad habits. Many of those who regularly take laxatives, health salts and so on fall into this third category.

No medicine should ever be taken regularly for more than five days unless it has been prescribed or recommended by a doctor.

MEDICINES THAT GO 'OFF'

Drugs may deteriorate when stored, particularly if stored in the damp or in direct sunlight, in extremes of heat or of cold. Some drugs when they deteriorate simply become less effective. Others turn into entirely different products – and can, therefore, be exceptionally dangerous.

To minimize the risk of deterioration medicines should be kept in closed containers away from the hazards I've outlined above. If your bathroom becomes very damp it may be better to keep your (locked) medicine cabinet in some other room.

And to minimize the risk of taking a deteriorated medicine always throw medicines away when the expiry date suggests that they should be thrown away. In general it is a good idea to keep the home medicine cabinet clear of all products except the ones I list on p. 193 as being suitable for keeping in store. Even those products should be replaced every six months or so.

THE PREGNANT WOMAN AND MEDICINES

The horror of the thalidomide story is still in the minds of most people but I never fail to be amazed at the number of pregnant women who take medicines. Many seem to think that home medicines are harmless. They are not. Even ordinary antacids, the ones used for indigestion, may cause problems if taken by pregnant women. As may aspirin tablets.

And it is not only medicines that are swallowed that can cause problems. The substance podophyllin applied to the skin is not normally absorbed, but changes in body physiology during pregnancy can mean that when podophyllin is applied to warts around the anus or vagina of a pregnant woman the unborn baby can be damaged.

It is undoubtedly a fact that many congenital defects are caused by drugs. It is also a fact that as yet we don't know which drugs cause which problems. The safest course is for pregnant women to avoid taking or using any home medicine. If they need some treatment then they should see a doctor and make sure that he knows that they are pregnant. The doctor can then at least ensure that the safest available product is used.

Exactly the same applies to women who are breast feeding. Mother's milk contains the drugs that she is taking and the newly born baby may suffer if the mother uses medicines unwisely.

PART 2

CHOOSING A MEDICINE
swallow it, chew it or rub it on?

Medicines are available in many different forms. Sometimes the same substance will be available as a tablet, a mixture, a suppository or a cream. Choosing the right way to take a medicine can be as important as choosing the right medicine.

There are several criteria to be used when making a selection.

Firstly, if a drug can be applied locally then it should be. The risks involved when a drug is taken orally are usually greater than when it is applied to the skin, for example. So, if an infected wound can be encouraged to heal with a superficial dressing the patient will have avoided the potential risks associated with taking tablets by mouth and exposing the entire bodily system to the action of a powerful drug.

Secondly, the choice of a drug may be affected by convenience. There isn't any point at all in having a bottle of medicine in the bathroom cabinet and suffering from indigestion in a traffic queue miles from home. However good the medicine is it won't work unless you take it. So, a box of antacid tablets may be more effective in those circumstances than a bottle of medicine because you'll carry the tablets with you – they're more convenient.

Thirdly, there are some types of presentation which make medicines particularly suitable for specific problems. An ointment, for example, may be just right for a very dry and crusty skin condition. A gargle or mouthwash may be the best way to alleviate discomfort in the mouth or throat and an inhalant may be the most effective way to deal with a stuffed-up nose. Choosing the right form in which to take a drug obviously depends, therefore, upon knowing what part of your body you're treating. An inhalant will be likely to alleviate headaches due to catarrh but it won't do much to help headaches caused by poor lighting at work.

To help make it easier to decide whether or not a liniment is likely to be more useful than a suppository, or a tablet better than a lozenge,

I have prepared a list of all the commonly used ways of preparing and offering medicines. Read through the list below and then use it as a guide when choosing the right medicine.

CHOOSING A MEDICINE – QUICK GUIDE

For a condition which involves the skin use an application, collodion, cream, gel, ointment, paint, paste or poultice.

For a condition involving the muscles use a balm, liniment, rub or rubefacient.

For a condition involving the mouth or throat use a gargle, insufflation, lozenge or mouthwash.

For a condition involving the lower bowel use an enema or suppository.

For a condition involving the vagina use a pessary.

For a condition which involves the body generally or which requires a medicine to be taken orally, use a cachet, capsule, elixir, granules, injection, mixture, pill, powder or tablet.

aerosol   solid or liquid particles of medicament suspended in a fine spray or mist.

application   any liquid or semi-liquid preparation which is applied to the skin.

balm   an aromatic ointment that is used to help heal a wound or to soothe pain. Balms are commonly used in the treatment of rheumatism.

cachet   a wafer or capsule which contains a medical substance.

capsule   a small soluble container which dissolves in the body releasing the medicine that is contained within it – usually in powder form. The two halves of a capsule are often coloured separately.

collodion   a clear, sticky liquid used to hold wounded edges together, keep dressings in place and seal sterile wounds. If medicaments are dissolved in a collodion their contact with the skin is prolonged.

cream   a medical substance with the consistency of the oily part of milk. Creams spread easier than ointments which tend to leave the skin sticky.

dusting powder   a fine powder which is shaken on to the body like talcum powder.

elixir   a sweetened aromatic preparation of a soluble medicinal substance. Elixirs are given 'miracle' properties by those with an interest in their sale.

emollient   an application rubbed on to the body to help soften and relax it.

emulsion   a mixture of two immiscible liquids, one dispersed throughout the other in small droplets.

enema   a solution designed for introduction into the rectum, either to promote evacuation of the bowel contents or to introduce food or medicine or X-ray material.

gargle   a solution for rinsing the mouth and throat.

gel   a jelly-like material.

granules   medicinal pellets which may be taken with or without water.

inhalation   a preparation designed to be drawn into the lungs. If you fill a bowl with boiling water, cover your head with a towel and breathe in the steam rising from the bowl through your nostrils you are inhaling water vapour. (This can help catarrh, etc.)

injection   the introduction of a liquid into the body. Injections can be into muscles, tissues or directly into blood vessels. Strictly speaking an enema is inserted by injection.

insufflation   a powder, vapour or gas designed to be blown into a body cavity – for example, the mouth and throat. Problems can occur if the patient blows back!

linctus   a syrupy medicine designed to be licked up with the tongue.

liniment   an oily liquid preparation to be rubbed on to the skin.

lotion   a liquid preparation for bathing a part of the body.

lozenge   a medicated troche. A troche is a dry, solid, medicated mass intended to be held in the mouth and slowly dissolved in the saliva. It was originally shaped like a diamond.

mixture   a medicinal preparation of two or more ingredients mixed together. Some manufacturers put dozens of different ingredients into their mixtures but frequently none of the ingredients are included in worthwhile quantities.

mouthwash   see **gargle**.

ointment   a semi-solid preparation for external application to the body which may contain a medicinal substance, e.g. an antihistamine, or an antibiotic. Ointments are greasier, stickier and messier than creams but can be useful on very dry, crusty skin.

paint   an external medicament which is put on with a brush – like any other paint!

paste   a semi-solid preparation, usually applied to the skin. Pastes are firmer than ointments.

pessary   an instrument placed inside the vagina to support the uterus, or a medicated vaginal suppository.

pill   a convenient way to serve up small doses of medicine in a suitable size for swallowing. Pills were originally prepared by hand, the chemist rolling the substance between his fingers with the movement that people use when playing with small pieces of plasticine.

potion   a large dose of liquid medicine. One that needs to be drunk rather than simply taken on a spoon.

poultice   a soft pulpy mass placed hot upon the skin as a counter-irritant to soothe a sore or inflamed part of the body. A hot-water bottle is probably just as good but it's nowhere near as much fun.

powder   a lot of tiny particles obtained by grinding a solid mass. Chemists used to use a mortar and pestle to make powders. (The mortar is the bowl.)

rub   a substance suitable for rubbing on to the skin (see **liniment** and **rubefacient**).

rubefacient   a substance that reddens and irritates the skin.

shake lotion   a convenient way of applying powder to the skin. The water in which the powder is suspended evaporates, cooling and soothing the skin, and the powder is left behind. Obviously it needs to be shaken before use. Calamine lotion is a good example.

solution   an evenly distributed solid available in liquid form.

spirit   a volatile or distilled liquid.

spray   a liquid which is available as a mist – a lot of tiny droplets.

suppository   a medicated solid mass of suitable size and consistency for inserting into a body cavity other than the mouth, e.g. vagina or rectum or urethra. Pessaries are suppositories which are placed inside the vagina.

tablet   a small amount of a drug compressed or moulded into shape by machine and containing a fixed amount of active ingredient. A tablet may be coated with various substances to conceal the taste or to delay its disintegration and absorption. Most modern pills are, in fact, tablets.

vapour rub   a substance for rubbing on to the skin which gives off a vapour and smells medicinal!

CHOOSING A MEDICINE
what sort of drug is it?

Medicine bottles often contain words like 'analgesic', 'expectorant' and 'purgative'. These and many other words are used to categorize products and throughout the following sections the same terms will recur. To avoid repeating definitions in the text and to help medicine buyers confused by jargon on labels and advertisements I have compiled an easy reference guide to the terms most commonly used by pharmacists, doctors and manufacturers.

I should perhaps point out that these definitions are not intended to be suitable for students of pharmacology!

anaesthetic a product that dulls the senses. For home use this invariably means a cream or spray which helps control irritation or pain.

analgesic a painkiller.

anorectic a drug that reduces the appetite. Clearly most slimming drugs fall into this category.

antacid something that counteracts or opposes the action of an acid. Antacids are usually prescribed for the relief of indigestion pains which may be exacerbated by the excessive production or availability of stomach acid.

antibiotic a chemical product which destroys living organisms. Antibiotics intended for use by mouth have to be prescribed by a doctor but there are creams, ointments and so on containing antibiotics which are available for home use.

anticholinergic a drug which interferes with the process whereby nervous impulses are passed through the body. They are sometimes used in the prevention of motion sickness, for example.

anti-emetic a product designed to prevent vomiting.

antihistamine   a substance which counteracts the effects of 'histamine', a chemical which is released within the body automatically when tissues are injured but which itself has unwanted effects. Reddening of the skin which occurs after a sting is caused by the production of histamine. An antihistamine drug can prevent that reaction developing.

anti-inflammatory   a drug which helps oppose inflammatory processes within the body. Inflammation can be caused by injury or infection and usually involves heat, redness, swelling and pain. An anti-inflammatory drug can help control those symptoms.

antiperspirant   a product which prevents sweating – for example, by blocking the pores in the skin.

antipyretic   something which helps bring down a fever or temperature. Aspirin has an antipyretic action.

antiseptic   a substance which destroys small organisms which may harm living tissues (see **disinfectant**).

antispasmodic   a drug which helps stop spasms. Muscle spasms can be a cause of pain, and an antispasmodic may therefore effectively prevent or relieve pain.

anxiolytic   a drug designed to help an anxious or worried patient. Effective anxiolytics usually need to be obtained on prescription.

aperient   a gentle laxative or fairly mild 'opening' medicine.

astringent   strictly speaking an astringent is something that prevents a discharge of any kind. Substances which stop bleeding may be astringents.

cathartic   a purgative or laxative. Something which helps to empty the bowels.

caustic   a substance which can burn and destroy.

cough suppressant   a substance which actually helps a patient stop coughing. Some cough medicines are not, in fact, designed to do this (see **expectorant**).

decongestant   usually means something which helps to relieve congestion or stuffiness in the nose and sinuses.

deodorant a product designed to remove (or prevent) unwanted body smells. A deodorant may contain a disinfectant (intended to destroy organisms which might otherwise break down human sweat and in the process produce a nasty smell) and/or a perfume designed to disguise unpleasant smells.

disinfectant a substance which destroys small organisms which may produce infection and harm living tissue. The word 'disinfectant' is usually kept for products which are used on inanimate objects which need to be kept clean (dirty sheets may be washed in a disinfectant), whereas the word 'antiseptic' is usually kept for products used on the human body (mouthwashes, lotions, creams and so on). However, this distinction is not always followed and the two words are often used by home medicine manufacturers as though they were interchangeable. Just to make matters even more confused there are manufacturers who claim that their products contain antiseptics and disinfectants. For practical purposes the words antiseptic and disinfectant are interchangeable.

diuretic a product which increases the flow of urine. By increasing the rate at which water is excreted from the body a diuretic may help reduce ankle swelling or other signs of fluid retention.

expectorant a medicine which helps a patient bring up sputum. It works by liquefying secretions which exist or by encouraging the production of fluids which will dilute secretions.

germicide an agent that destroys small organisms. For practical purposes as far as home medicines are concerned germicide is interchangeable with antiseptic and disinfectant.

hypnotic a drug that helps produce sleep. Powerful hypnotics are only available on prescription and mild hypnotics probably rely heavily on the placebo effect (see p.32).

keratolytic a powerful substance used to destroy unwanted skin (such as warts and corns) but which can damage good, healthy skin.

laxative a medicine which helps empty the bowels. Laxative, purgative and cathartic all mean the same thing.

medicated this word is used by many manufacturers as though it automatically improved the quality of any product. It simply means that the product concerned contains a substance which has medicinal properties. For example, sticking plasters which are treated with anti-septics are described as 'medicated' as are sweets which contain minute quantities of substances which have mild medicinal qualities.

preservative   labels on medicine bottles often list ingredients des-cribed as preservatives. These substances do exactly the same job as the preservatives added to foodstuffs – they help stop the product going bad.

prophylactic   strictly speaking a prophylactic is anything which helps prevent disease. In everyday language, however, a prophylactic often means a condom. This specialized definition has some validity if you regard pregnancy as a disease.

purgative   a medicine which helps empty the bowels (see **laxative**). The British sometimes seem to be obsessed with the behaviour of their bowels and the number of available words which can be used to describe drugs which have an effect on 'stubborn' bowels seems to illustrate this obsession rather well.

sedative   a drug which has a calming effect. Most sedatives also cause drowsiness. Powerful sedatives are only available on prescription.

stimulant   a substance which excites all or part of the human body. Caffeine is a stimulant which has a general effect on human beings.

tranquillizer   a medicine which has a calming effect. Tranquillizers are supposed to cause less drowsiness than sedatives but in practical terms this difference is usually rather slight.

vasodilator   a chemical which opens up the blood vessels and thereby encourages the flow of blood to the tissues. Products designed for use by patients with chilblains may be described as vasodilators. There is much contradictory evidence about the effectiveness of drugs in this category.

BUYING A HOME MEDICINE

Do check the price of the product you are buying with comparable alternatives. New, well-advertised products are inevitably more expensive than products that are not advertised. You can pay twice as much for a well-known brand name as for a product which contains exactly the same ingredients. Products marked BP or BPC have to be prepared to official standards and are often cheaper than products with well-known names. New and wonderful products usually contain old drugs in new packaging; most are simply variations on existing themes.

USING A HOME MEDICINE

Do not store a home medicine for more than six months. Throw out discoloured tablets and mixtures which do not return to their original colour and consistency after a shake. Do not open capsules or crush tablets which are not designed to be crushed. Never use unlabelled medicines. If you have to dispose of old drugs either take them along to your pharmacist or throw them down the lavatory.

Make sure that when you buy a home medicine you know when to take it and how much to take. If you are buying a liquid medicine ask the pharmacist for a measuring spoon. The small print on the side of a medicine bottle is often very important.

AVOIDING DANGER

Don't buy or use home medicines if you are taking prescribed medicines, if you suffer from a long-term disorder or if you are pregnant or breast feeding. Never use a home medicine regularly. Home medicines are designed for the treatment and alleviation of acute problems not chronic ones. Knowing when *not* to use a home medicine is probably more important than knowing when to use one. Don't take extra doses of home medicines if the recommended doses don't work. Mae West is reported to have said that 'too much of a good thing is wonderful'. Whatever else she was talking about it wasn't medicines. Don't mix home medicines, don't give adult doses to children and *always* keep medicines in a lockable cupboard or well out of reach of children.

WHEN YOU GO TO THE DOCTOR . . .

. . . tell him if you have already tried to treat yourself without success. For example, if you have indigestion and you've tried a particular antacid then tell him. Otherwise you may find yourself leaving the surgery with a prescription for exactly the same product. Remember that self-medication is a supplement to medical care not a substitute or competitor.

TWELVE RULES FOR SAFETY

1 **Always** read and follow any instructions and warnings provided by the manufacturer. **Never** exceed the recommended dose.

2 **Always** keep medicines – even apparently harmless ones – out of the reach of children.

3 **Don't** take home medicines if you are taking anything prescribed by a doctor – unless you have his permission.

4 **Never** continue with home treatment for more than five days.

5 If you are in doubt about how to use a medicine **ask** the pharmacist.

6 If you are taking a medicine **don't** drink alcohol.

7 Some home medicines cause drowsiness – so **beware**!

8 Pregnant women should **never** take home medicines unless they've consulted a doctor first.

9 **Don't** use old medicines. Buy in small quantities and replace stocks every six months or so.

10 **Never** use old medicines if you aren't sure what they are. Anything without a proper label should be thrown away.

11 If you intend travelling outside northern Europe see your travel agent or doctor to check up on what vaccinations or medicines you may need to take.

12 If you develop any unusual or persistent symptoms on returning from a trip abroad get in touch with your doctor straight away. **Don't** try treating disorders which may have been contracted in foreign countries by yourself.

HOW TO USE THE DIRECTORY

The home medicines in this directory are all listed according to the symptoms they are designed to treat. Look up the specific symptom you are interested in in the index at the back and you will be directed to the relevant section of the directory. When compiling this directory I had to assume that readers would know what symptoms they wanted to treat – indigestion, backache or whatever.

Some symptoms will inevitably lead to several sections. If you look up 'itching', for example, you will be referred to allergies, skin disorders and worms. **If after consulting the various sections you are in any way uncertain about the diagnosis then a doctor should always be consulted.**

To facilitate cross reference I have kept similar types of problems within the same main section. In the section 'Colds and flu, coughs and sore throats', for example, I have listed all treatments for catarrh, coughs, fever and sore throats since these symptoms often occur together and the treatment for one is likely to be related to the treatment for another.

THE DIRECTORY

ACNE, SPOTS, PIMPLES AND BOILS

Human skin, is, if I may say so without appearing impertinent, brilliantly designed, It can withstand tremendous amounts of pressure, it stretches to accommodate the shape of the bones and organs within it and, perhaps most amazing of all, it can regenerate when it's damaged. Cells which wear out are replaced automatically and skin can protect itself against the sun by increasing the deposit of melanin cells near to the surface. It keeps itself moist by secreting a substance called sebum from sebaceous cells and even contains hair cells which, although rather unnecessary today, were originally designed to help keep the human organism warm when the winter turned nasty.

It is perhaps inevitable, therefore, that occasionally things will go slightly wrong. One particularly common problem, affecting nearly all of us as we pass through our adolescent years, is acne.

Acne is a disorder of the sebaceous glands within the skin, the glands which produce sebum. Without sebum our skin would be dry and it would crack on bending. With sebum the skin is supple and elastic. Problems arise when the channel through which sebum reaches the surface becomes blocked. The dead and useless cells forming the blockage can turn black producing what is commonly known as a 'blackhead'. If the blocked gland at the base of the blockage becomes infected a reddened, inflamed spot may develop and eventually pus may start leaking out on to the surface of the skin.

There really is not much difference between an infected acne spot and a pimple; and a boil is simply a rather large infected spot. Where two or three infected spots are gathered together in one small area with deep tissue involvement the result is described as a carbuncle.

Antiseptic creams and liquids (see also pp.97–8)
Many of the products sold for the treatment of acne contain antiseptics (substances which destroy microorganisms). *Germolene Antiseptic Ointment* is recommended for the treatment of spots as well as the treatment of cuts, scratches, grazes, blisters and rough skin! The manufacturers of *TCP Liquid Antiseptic* claim that their product is 'today's most used spot treatment'. *Torbetol Liquid* consists of three antiseptics: cetrimide, hexachlorophene and benzalkonium bromide.

Spotoway is available as a tincture or cream and contains 'powerful, hospital-proved antiseptics' together with 'natural, herbal preparations to soothe and cool inflamed and infected skin'. *Betadine Skin Cleanser* and *Betadine Skin Cleanser Foam* both contain a type of iodine. A main active ingredient of *Swiss Bio-Facial* is chlorhexidine which is an antiseptic. *Cuxson Gerrard Boil Treatment* consists of plasters bearing hexachlorophene or aminacrine ointments; both of these are antiseptics, and *Sevilan Acne Cream* contains among other things decamethylen-bis-4-amino-chinaldinium chloride which is also an antiseptic.

The only problem with all these treatments is that many spots are not infected or infectious and therefore an antiseptic which is designed to treat or prevent infection is not really suitable. Once acne spots have become widely infected then antibiotic therapy is probably necessary (see p.62).

Soaps

Special soaps are available for preventing the development of spots and pimples or for treating already infected skin.

Examples of these are *Clearasil Soap* which contains sulphur and *Cidal Soap* which contains irgasan, an antiseptic.

Prolonged use (more than five days) of any medicated soap cannot be recommended, since continued use can cause allergy rashes.

Keratolytics

These are substances which help to clear away dead skin cells, literally peeling away blackheads to unblock the pores. Resorcinol is a basic ingredient of a number of preparations such as *Acnil, Avrogel, Clearasil Cream Medication (Skin Tinted* and *White), DDD Lotion, Eskamel, Medac Acne Cream, pHiso-Ac, Vanispot* and *Wigglesworth Acne Cream*.

Salicylic acid is another keratolytic that is present in *Avrogel, Clearasil Cleansing Lotion, Dermaclear* and *DDD Lotion*.

A third keratolytic substance, benzoyl peroxide, is obtainable as *Benoxyl 5* and *Benoxyl 10*, both either plain or with sulphur, *Dry Clear Acne Lotion, Panoxyl 5 Acne Gel* and *Panoxyl 10 Acne Gel, Quinoderm* and *Vanair*.

You can buy non-branded versions of some of these basic ingredients.

Resorcinol is available as *Compound Resorcinol Ointment BPC* or *Resorcinol and Sulphur Paste BPC*. Salicylic acid is available as *Salicylic Acid and Sulphur Cream BPC*. *Zinc Sulphide Lotion BNF* is also available.

Abrasives

Some of the substances used in proprietary acne preparations work by removing the blockage or blackheads which are sealing up the skin's sebaceous glands. It is possible to do much the same thing merely by rubbing the skin with something rough – removing the blackheads and dead cells by physical rather than chemical means.

To assist in this process you can buy a non-medicated cleansing sponge called a *Buf-puf* or a paste called *Brasivol* which contains graded particles of aluminium oxide. You can buy *Brasivol* in three grades: fine, medium and coarse.

However, you don't *have* to buy anything special. You can get exactly the same effect by using a rough flannel, a loofah or a fairly soft nail-brush. Individual blackheads can be removed by being squeezed out. This does at least stop the blackheads becoming infected. It is best to remove blackheads after washing the face with hot water and although you can use your fingernails you can buy special devices for squeezing out blackheads or 'comedones' as they are known in the trade. Ask for a comedo expressor. One word of warning, however: do not try squeezing infected blackheads – you'll probably make things worse.

Ultraviolet light (see also p.161)

Ultraviolet lamps can help ease the problem by encouraging skin peeling. As the skin peels so the blocked ducts are cleared. Ordinary sunlight produces exactly the same effect, of course, and so it is wise for the acne sufferer to get as much sun as possible. Artificial lamps should be used with great care and instructions followed to the letter. There isn't much point in replacing acne with burns.

A 'magic' solution

Heath and Heather manufacture *Blood Purifying Tablets* and a *Blood Purifying Mixture* said to 'assist in clearing the blood of impurities in the case of boils, pimples, etc.'.

The mixture contains, among other things, arctium lappa (once used as a diuretic and also known in common circles as the dried root of the Great Burdock but that doesn't sound half so grand and scientific does it?) and senna (a very effective laxative).

Rather surprisingly the tablets do not contain the same ingredients as the mixture. In a tablet you get such delights as buckbean (also known rather aptly as bogbean) which is a purgative and can cause vomiting, although in larger doses than contained in the tablets.

I suppose the theory is that since constipation is a cause of spots (and I used to have an aunt who swore that all spots were caused by recalcitrant bowels) a cure for the constipation will also prove to be a cure for the spots.

Avoiding acne

Although there have been many theories about the cause of acne there is not much you can do to prevent yourself developing spots. It has in the past been said that chocolate, peanuts and fatty or milky foods in general can cause spots. I don't really think that there is any scientific evidence supporting any of these theories, although they may be coincidental.

There are hormonal and hereditary reasons for the skin changes which result in the development of acne and it is the hormonal reasons (related to the level of sex hormones) which result in the high incidence of acne in adolescents. It is this hormonal influence which is responsible for the common phrase 'you'll grow out of it'. For most young sufferers that really is the last thing they want to hear. They're worried about what they look like *now*, not what they're going to look like in ten or twenty years' time.

It is probably worthwhile pointing out to teenage girls who suffer from spots that face creams which are sometimes used to cover up blackheads and acne lesions may in fact make things worse by blocking up the ducts leading out of the sebaceous glands. Even antiseptic creams can do this, thereby making the condition they are intended to treat far worse.

Boils

There really isn't anything much you can do about boils. It certainly is not a good idea to smear them with antiseptic creams. Nor is it sensible to try squeezing them. Both these courses are likely to result in a bigger, longer-lasting boil. It's far more sensible to put a warm compress on top of the boil (or just hold a hot-water bottle near to it). With warmth the boil will burst quicker and the pain and mess will be over quicker.

If a boil doesn't come to a head after five days then see a doctor. Similarly seek advice if the boil is in a particularly unbearable spot (in your nose or ear or on your bottom) and you want it lanced before then. If you get a crop of boils then it is worth seeking a doctor's advice. You or some member of the family may be carrying the infective organism which is responsible for the boils. I once treated a family in which the father kept getting boils and the son needed treatment with an antibiotic. The bug that was causing the father's boils was hiding out in the son's nose without causing him any ill effects at all.

When to see a doctor

Your doctor cannot do much that you can't do yourself for simple blackheads that haven't got infected. But if you have an unsightly crop of red, infected spots on your face or back a course of antibiotic therapy may prove helpful or even essential if you are to avoid future scarring. Most doctors prescribe antibiotics for several months when they're needed and it is important for patients to be aware of the fact that little improvement can be expected for the first month or two.

Conclusion

It probably isn't worthwhile trying to do anything about the odd spot or two. They'll go away by themselves if left alone – even if they become infected.

If you suffer from a lot of blackheads try to get out into the sun as often as possible and either use an abrasive or wash regularly with a coarse flannel or brush. A keratolytic may help to clear out blocked pores.

If spots become red, inflamed and swollen and do not clear up in five days see your own doctor.

ALLERGIES

The boy with hay fever, the girl who can't go near dogs without developing a rash, the woman who can't put her hands into detergent and the man who develops nasty-looking red blotches if he eats strawberries, all have allergies.

As is the case with so many symptoms, when you have an allergic reaction it is because your body is trying to protect itself. The symptoms (itching, sneezing, watering eyes or nose or a red rash) simply mean that the body's defence mechanisms have overdone things. Allergy reactions are simply immune reactions that have gone wrong.

When an allergy reaction is due to something that has been swallowed (such as a food or a drug) then the whole body will be affected. Usually there will be a red, itchy rash over most areas. So, the reaction of someone allergic to penicillin will be very similar to the reaction of someone allergic to lobster.

When an allergy reaction is due to something which has been in contact with one part of the body, then the symptoms are likely to be more specific. Hay fever sufferers commonly have itching eyes, a runny nose and bouts of sneezing because the pollen only affects the areas around the nasal mucosa. Women who are allergic to eye makeup will only develop puffiness and itchiness around their eyes. Men allergic to oils will develop symptoms on the parts of their bodies which have been in contact with oil. The reaction we show after being stung or bitten by an insect is an allergic reaction. The reaction is to poison, saliva or some other substance left in the body by the insect.

Most allergies are annoying rather than dangerous. Obviously dangerous allergies (which may be heralded by a really severe reaction sometimes accompanied by breathlessness and other serious problems) need medical help. Less serious allergies can be dealt with without professional advice.

The basic weapon against an allergy reaction is an antihistamine. Before I go any further I must warn you that an antihistamine is a substance which has been described as a drug which turns a sneeze into a yawn. Every year there are new antihistamines brought out which manufacturers claim cause less drowsiness. Within months it is usually perfectly clear that the new 'wonder' drugs can cause drowsiness. The best thing to do is to experiment with antihistamines until you find the one that causes you least drowsiness. Car drivers should be particularly aware of this complication and of the fact that alcohol makes the drowsiness worse.

Having said that, it is important to make it clear immediately that antihistamines are extremely effective. They ought to be: when a trigger produces an allergy reaction, the body's defence mechanisms include the production of a chemical called histamine. It is this substance which produces the irritation and rash which so often accompany an allergy reaction.

Some of the best-known antihistamine drugs are *Actidil*, *Anthisan*, *Benadryl*, *Daneral SA*, *Dimotane*, *Fabahistin*, *Haymine*, *Histryl*, *Optimine*, *Periactin*, *Phenergan*, *Piriton* and *Pro-Actidil*. Each product has its fans. Prices vary considerably and I suggest that if you're experimenting, you start with the cheapest.

Incidentally, dark glasses (see p.165) may relieve some of the eye symptoms associated with hay fever. I do not recommend the use of antihistamine eye drops unless the drops have been prescribed by a doctor.

Nor do I recommend that you buy nose drops or sprays (such as *Antistin*, *Fenox*, *Hayphryn* and *Otrivine*) without a doctor's advice unless you restrict your use of them to five days or less, because the nasal mucosa is very delicate and can easily be damaged.

Creams which are recommended for the local treatment of allergy reactions often contain an antihistamine, calamine and possibly a local anaesthetic as well. These products are discussed in **Stings** p.160.

BABY PROBLEMS

Some products sold for the treatment of baby problems are either superfluous or potentially harmful or both. If a baby's problem persists or proves worrying then consult an expert. Read one of the many excellent volumes on baby care to ensure that you know what signs and symptoms to look out for.

The treatment of problems in older children is usually the same as the treatment of the same problems in adults except that dosages will differ. Always study the manufacturer's recommended dosages before giving any medicines.

Cough and cold remedies

The following products for baby's coughs and colds are available: *Baby Cough Syrup, Buttercup Baby Cough Linctus, Cox's Children's Cherry Cough Linctus, Famel Children's Cough Linctus, Galloway's Junior Cough Linctus, Willocare Junior Expectorant* and *Wright's Baby Cough Linctus* (see p.78).

I do not recommend any of these products which are unlikely to have any useful action in that in my opinion they do not contain sufficient medicament to effect a cure.

If a baby's cough does not resolve after five days or if the baby has difficulty in breathing then consult a doctor. If a baby has the snuffles or seems congested, he may be helped if a kettle is boiled in the same room. Children over the age of six can, if necessary, be treated with reduced doses of adult mixtures. It is as practicable to decide on the dosage according to the child's weight as on his age. Thus, a four-stone child should be given approximately half the normal adult dose.

Diarrhoea

A child who has diarrhoea should be treated in the same way as anyone else (see p.106). A baby with diarrhoea may need medical attention earlier, since it is possible for a baby to become dehydrated remarkably quickly. I do not recommend any special mixtures. *Child's Diarrhoea Mixture* contains, among other things, clioquinol which is discussed on p.110. *Paediatric Kaolin Mixture BPC* can be given in a dose of 5 ml to children under the age of one year and 10 ml to children over the age of one year. The dose can be repeated at four-hourly intervals, but it is more likely to make the parents feel better than the child.

Feeding

Breast milk is obviously best for most babies since it was formulated by an expert and contains many valuable constituents not available in other types of milk (for example, a baby who is breast fed will be protected from infections by his mother's antibodies).

However, it is a fact that for one reason or another many young mothers are not willing or able to feed their babies themselves, and there are a number of perfectly adequate replacements for breast milk.

Recommended proprietary milk foods for infants under six months of age include *Babymilk Plus, Cow & Gate Premium Babyfood, Cow & Gate V Formula, Ostermilk Complete Formula, SMA* and *Gold Cap SMA*.

I do not recommend *National Dried Milk* for infants under six months of age.

Gripe mixtures

Most babies have wind or indigestion occasionally. Usually the disorder can be treated without any medicine.

Sodium bicarbonate (see p.124) is included in many gripe remedies. It is a constituent of the following products: *Atkinson and Barker's Infant Gripe Mixture, Baby Gripe Mixture, Boots Gripe Mixture, Dinneford's Gripe Mixture, Fennings' Gripe Mixture, Gould's Gripe Mixture, Maws Gripe Mixture, Nurse Harvey's Gripe Mixture* and *Woodward's Gripe Water*. Some of these products also contain alcohol.

Calmic Gripe Mixture contains dimethicone (see p.125) which is intended to help relieve wind.

Merbentyl, a product often prescribed by doctors for griping pains in babies, contains dicyclomine hydrochloride which is an antispasmodic. Children under one year should be given 2.5 ml before feeds. Above one year, the dose can be increased to 5 ml up to three times a day.

Ovol Colic Drops contain both dimethicone and dicyclomine.

Any of these products can help and doctors often prescribe, as I have said, dicyclomine hydrochloride for griping pains, but these substances should only be used when the diagnosis is certain. Incidentally, babies who get wind during and after feeding are often being fed improperly – a young mother who cannot obtain advice from a female relative should consult her doctor or health visitor.

Persistent griping pains should be investigated by a doctor anyway.

Nappy rash

To stop a baby developing a nappy rash, ensure that wet nappies are removed as soon as possible and washed and rinsed thoroughly. Disposable nappies are expensive but safe and convenient. Tightly fitting rubber or plastic pants help to encourage the development of a rash, nude crawling prevents it.

There are several useful treatments for nappy rash. Zinc and castor oil ointment is often all that is needed. It is available as *Zinc and Castor Oil Ointment BPC* or as *Zincast Baby Cream*, and there are other branded products available.

Dimethicone Cream BPC may help, and there are a number of branded products which also contain silicone, a water repellent substance which can provide effective protection and prevent the development of a rash. These include *Boots Nappy Cream, Neo Baby Cream, Steedman's Nappy Cream* and *Vasogen*. Unfortunately, *Boots, Neo* and *Steedman's* all contain an antiseptic which may well be unnecessary and which may cause irritation, possibly potentially harmful, although medical opinion is divided on this point. *Maws Baby Lotion, Moores Baby Cream, Natusan Baby Cream, Savlon Babycare Cream* or *Woodward's Baby Cream* also contain antiseptics and *Natusan* contains boric acid which should be avoided since it can be toxic even when only applied to the skin.

Any nappy rash which persists after treatment for a week or ten days or which seems to be getting worse despite treatment can be treated more effectively by a doctor.

Pain relievers

Paracetamol is a popular basis for children's pain relieving remedies. The following products contain paracetamol: *Calpol, De Witt's Placidex, Febrilix, Fennings' Children's Cooling Powders, Hush, Panets Baby Syrup* and *Pirisol Junior Pain Tablets*. These products should be taken according to the manufacturer's instructions. Paracetamol can, however, be purchased in non-branded form as *Paediatric Paracetamol Elixir BPC*. Children under one year should be given 5 ml at a time. Children between 1 and 5 years can be given 10 ml at a time.

Paracetamol is preferred to aspirin since it can be produced in elixir or medicine form. Aspirin is only available as tablets in such products as *Angiers Junior Aspirin, Junior Disprin* and *Parkinsons Children's Aspirin Tablets* (see also p.134).

Teething remedies
Teething preparations are largely useless. When applied to gums or to emerging teeth, they are quickly washed away in the saliva. Products available include *Baby Gum Lotion, Dentinox Teething Gel, Dentinox Teething Liquid, Steedman's Teething Jelly* and *Woodward's Teething Balm,* and although a mild painkiller is probably more useful it might be worthwhile trying *Dentinox* and *Woodward's* because both contain a local anaesthetic.

Miscellaneous
There are many products for the prevention or treatment of other illnesses or problems in babies and children. I do not recommend any of them. A baby or child who needs a medicine other than of the type I've mentioned here needs a doctor. Never take any chances with babies or children – always ask for professional advice if you are in any doubt about the diagnosis or treatment.

BACKACHE (see also **Pain** p.134)
More than half of all adults have backache at some time or another. People in their forties and fifties are most at risk and back pains are said to cost Britain about £200 million a year in lost work and sickness payments. In a single year 1½ million people will visit their doctors for treatment for backache and on any one day 50,000 British men and women will be off work with backache.

There are many reasons why people suffer from backache. If the pain follows a fall then clearly urgent investigations need to be done to exclude a fracture. More commonly backache follows heavy lifting, heavy work in the garden or a long period spent sitting in an uncomfortable position.

Treatment for non-accidental backache consists of three things: heat, rest and pain relief.

A warm bath or a hot-water bottle (see p.141) will help relieve almost all muscular aches and pains whether caused by too much of the wrong kind of exercise or by tenseness and anxiety.

Rest is obviously vital. A few days in bed may sound daunting but the alternative may well be a few weeks in bed.

Pain relief can be obtained very effectively with simple analgesics such as aspirin or paracetamol. If you visit your doctor with a back-strain the chances are that he will tell you to go home and rest and that he will give you a prescription for paracetamol or aspirin.

If back pain is accompanied by pains in the legs there may be a slipped disc or nerve root irritation and a doctor's help may be needed. Similarly if pain persists for more than five days and shows no sign of abating then ask for help. Most doctors these days are happy for their patients to see qualified osteopaths.

Avoiding backache is obviously wiser than learning how to treat it and doing nothing to prevent it.

To avoid getting aches and pains in your back do not suddenly take up heavy exercise if you haven't done any physical work for years. Backaches are common in early spring when gardeners start digging over their vegetable patches.

If you have to pick up something heavy bend your knees and lift with your back kept straight.

Finally, learn to relax your muscles when you're sitting in the same position for long periods of time (see my book *Stress Control*).

BAD BREATH

Bad breath (known officially as halitosis) can be a most embarrassing and socially destructive problem. It is important to understand, however, that using a breath freshening perfume is not necessarily the right approach – just as it wasn't particularly logical for royal courtiers a century or two ago to use powerful perfumes to cover up the fact that they didn't bathe very often.

Bad breath can be caused by a number of soluble problems. Sinusitis, persistent catarrh, gingivitis and other dental problems can all be responsible for a malodorous mouth. A visit to the doctor or dentist may provide a permanent solution.

Meanwhile, if you want to paper over the cracks while you're waiting for more basic repair work to be done there are several alternative remedies available.

Antiseptic mouthwashes (such as *TCP* or *Oraldene*) may help by assisting in clearing up infections in the mouth and may, indeed, provide a permanent solution in some cases. Chlorophyll pills and tablets such as *Sweet-breaths* which contain a mixture of oils can provide a temporary solution. Regular tooth cleaning can help disguise bad breath as well as clearing away debris and preventing the development of further infection.

BREAST IMPROVERS
Many women are unhappy about the size of their breasts and would dearly like to find a way either to make them smaller or larger. There are to my knowledge no home remedies for those who would like their breasts to be smaller. The only solution available is to find a plastic surgeon. On the other hand for women who want to increase their breast size new remedies are often being introduced and promoted.

The best-known aid currently being sold is probably the *Aquamaid*. This consists of a device which enables a woman to splash cold water on to her breasts. The manufacturers naturally call it hydrotherapy. A similar result could probably be obtained by standing in a cold shower, dipping the breasts into a bowl full of cold water or allowing some loved one to throw cupfuls of water on to the offendingly small glands in the bath. There would almost certainly be some temporary increase in nipple size and possibly some increase in breast size but I am doubtful about the permanency of any effect obtained.

Food supplements such as lecithin, vitamin E and vitamin F are sold to help improve the quantity and quality of breast tissue. Massage creams containing vitamin E and vitamin F are advertised as helping to increase bust size. The manufacturers of the water device described above also make *Natural Vitamin E Cream* which they say will 'help breast tone and promote form and more prominent contours'. I am sceptical.

CHILBLAINS
Chilblains are common in Britain, but relatively rare in many other countries. It is our temperate, changeable weather that does it, for in countries where the weather is more predictable, chilblains are hardly known.

The best way to stop chilblains developing and the best way to make them go away is to keep warm. Since it is the extremities which are commonly affected, cosy socks and gloves are a must for chilblain sufferers. They should be loose so as not to impede the circulation. It is obviously more difficult to keep the tip of the nose and the lobes of the ears warm but these too can develop chilblains.

A chilblain is, in fact, nothing more than a spasm of the tiny vessels which provide the tissues with blood. Because of the cold, the blood vessels close up tightly. This is, in fact, a natural defence mechanism used by the body to retain heat – it is, unfortunately, one of those defence mechanisms which can cause problems.

The symptoms are well known to sufferers. There is pain, itching and swelling and the skin may change from bright red to blue. There may later be blistering and ulceration and if this happens a doctor's advice and help should be sought to avoid further damage.

Treatment is of two kinds: tablets and ointments.

Tablets usually contain drugs which are designed to help open up the blood vessels (vasodilators). These are of doubtful value, but occasionally seem to work.

Nicotinic acid is one possibly useful drug. *Nicotinic Acid Tablets BP* are available and should be taken in 100 mg doses three times a day.

Another tablet constituent is acetomenaphthone which is available together with nicotinic acid in *Amisyn, Boots Chilblain Tablets, Chilblain Treatment Dellipsoids D 27, GON tablets, Pernivit* and *Vitathone Chilblain Tablets*.

Creams and ointments include *Boots Chilblain Cream, Chilblain Cream, Samaritan Chilblain Cream, Scholl Chilblain Ointment, Vitathone Chilblain Cream* and *Willocare Chilblain Ointment*. Any of these substances may help increase cutaneous blood flow and the very act of rubbing something on may prove useful in stimulating the circulation.

It is not wise to put the part of the body with chilblains on it too near to a fire.

Finally, remember that chilblains are effectively nothing more than very early frostbite. They are best avoided by keeping warm all over in damp, cold weather and by making sure that the whole body is protected against the cold. Rubbing chilblains with snow, as some old wives suggest, is as silly as it sounds. There is, incidentally, one very simple way to improve the circulation in your hands: simply whirl your arms about using the same sort of movements that a bowler uses in cricket. Centrifugal forces push the blood down into the hands.

COLDS AND FLU, COUGHS AND SORE THROATS

The common cold and the almost equally common influenza are today responsible for most of the days off work and days off school taken by people all around the world. Despite the progress that has been made in many areas of medicine, doctors can still do very little about preventing colds or treating them. The scientific search for a cure for the common cold was started in 1926 by Dr Alphonse Dochez working in New York and in 1946 it was intensified when the British Medical Research Council set up a Common Cold Research Unit in Salisbury. Today, however, the man who helped set up the British unit admits that it is unlikely that any cure will ever be found. It seems, therefore, that we must learn to live with cold and respiratory tract infections and to cope with them as best as we can.

Many people seem confused by the terms 'cold' and 'flu' and use them indiscriminately. In fact, the symptoms of a common cold are far less fearsome than the symptoms of flu. The patient with a cold will usually complain of a streaming nose and of sneezing attacks. The patient with the more debilitating flu will, however, complain of sweating, headache, muscle aches and pains and a general feeling of great weakness. The patient with a cold can often struggle to work; the patient with flu will usually have great difficulty in dragging himself out of bed.

Both the common cold and the flu usually last for a week or so. Whether or not the flu or cold sufferer goes to work or stays at home depends upon several factors. It naturally depends upon just how bad the victim feels but it also depends on the type of work involved, the route to work and the feelings of other people at work.

Naturally, a man who works as a labourer on a building site will be better off at home if he has a really bad cold. The man who works alone in an office may be able to work fairly easily. The man whose job is twenty miles away will be less enthusiastic about going to work than the man who has to travel only a hundred yards. And the man who works in a busy office will be unpopular if he turns up!

By and large, children can usually give their mothers a good idea about whether or not they are fit to go to school themselves. The child with a cold should be fine for school as long as he is not sneezing too much, but the child with a high temperature and general muscle pains will need to be and want to be kept at home.

To sum up: the ordinary common cold (in case you've never had one) produces a swollen, inflamed nasal mucosa, with the result that the sufferer feels blocked up and has a runny nose. There is often an attendant sore throat, cough and headache together with a slight temperature and a collection of aches and pains. The flu sufferer will probably have a higher temperature and feel weaker.

The first thing to remember is that although you may not think so your body is reacting to a cold or flu virus for a very good reason. You have a temperature because your body is trying to kill off the invading germs and the aches and pains you feel should be telling you to take things easy.

Preventing colds and flu

There isn't anything really practicable you can do to prevent yourself getting a cold or an attack of influenza. Vaccinations were popular a year or two ago but now a large body of medical opinion believes that these do not make very much difference at all. Indeed some patients seem to get more colds after a vaccination. Tablets and capsules which are sold to prevent flu usually contain vitamins, although *Esobactulin Capsules* are said to contain special proteins designed to provide immunity for three months. I do not know of any independent evidence which supports this claim.

The only effective way to avoid catching colds is to keep away from people. Avoiding crowds you don't have to mix with is sensible enough but I don't suppose many people would want to go as far as the late Howard Hughes in their attempts to avoid germs – he even made his typist wear rubber gloves so that he wouldn't be contaminated when signing letters.

A considerable amount of research work has been done to investigate the claims made by a small number of eminent medical men that vitamin C stops people getting colds. The claims are true only in so far as it is correct that if you are deprived of vitamin C and develop scurvy (even a relatively mild form) then you will be more likely to catch a cold and to suffer badly from it. Anyone who is short of vitamin C needs to have the deficiency made good by a doctor.

If you have eaten a diet which has provided you with enough vitamin C (a diet which includes regular fruit and vegetables, for example) then extra vitamin C won't help you fight off a cold, suffer less or shake one off more speedily. A report in the *Journal of the American Medical Association* in 1979 showed that when Marine recruits were given doses of 2 gm of vitamin C a day they were not protected. That dose is a great deal higher than anything you would be likely to get from most of the proprietary medicines.

Despite the fact that, in my opinion, there is no convincing evidence to justify the claim, many manufacturers offer cold remedies containing vitamin C either as curatives or preventatives. Sometimes vitamin C seems to be thrown in with a whole host of other substances simply because it will look good on the packet.

The following products all contain vitamin C: *Anapax Cold Tablets, Beechams Powders with Hot Lemon, Boots Cold Relief Sachets, Boots Cold Tablets with Vitamin C, Cold Discs, Coldrex Powders, Coldrex Tablets, Cough Lem-Sip, Esocol Cold Treatment Tablets, Junior Lem-Sip* and *Lem-Sip*.

Fever, headaches and general aches and pains

Although it may not be easy to believe at the time, when you have a temperature and feel full of aches and pains your body is doing its best to protect itself against the invading infection. You have a temperature because your body is trying to kill off the invading germs and the aches and pains you suffer should be telling you to take it easy.

You can solve all these symptoms with simple aspirin or paracetamol (see p.134). Do remember, however, that even if the pills make you feel better you should resist the temptation to undertake heavy physical work straight away. Take it easy for a day or two and you'll get better quicker.

Catarrh, congestion and a runny nose

The mucosa inside your nose produces vast quantities of sticky mucus every day. This mucus traps dust particles as they enter the nose with each sniff of air. Mucus and dust are then usually swallowed. This is a normal, healthy process and needs no treatment.

When the process is interfered with the mucosa becomes inflamed and swollen and the mucus collects and perhaps gets infected. The symptoms may include a headache and a feeling of stuffiness.

Usually this problem will clear up in a few days. If it hasn't started to resolve after five days then a doctor's advice should be sought. While you're suffering there are many home medicines to choose from. They fall into three main categories. To begin with there are the drugs you swallow. Ephedrine, pseudoephedrine, phenylephrine and phenyl-propanolamine all help to cure wheezing and stuffiness. Unfortunately, these are powerful drugs and when given in large enough dosage to do any good (which to be honest they aren't in many home medicines) they can cause anxiety, restlessness, headaches and vomiting. They can also be very dangerous for people taking prescribed pills or for patients with heart disease. Atropine, belladonna and hyoscine are among the drugs used to dry up secretions. These can cause dryness, dizziness and sickness and can also affect the heart. The antihistamines (available in many different forms) are said to dry up secretions. Unfortunately, anti-histamines cause drowsiness and because of their drying effect they can help produce a worse infection in the long run.

The basic danger is a consequence of the fact that these powerful drugs don't just act on the nose or sinuses but have an effect through-out the body.

Two of the best known and most widely advertised products for catarrh are *Mu-Cron* and *Dō-Dō* – both available as tablets. *Mu-Cron Tablets* contain paracetamol, ipecacuanha, phenylpropanolamine hydrochloride and guaiphenesin. Paracetamol is a painkiller which is described at greater length on p.135; ipecacuanha when given in small doses is an expectorant which is particularly useful when the amount of sputum is slight; phenylpropanolamine hydrochloride is a decongest-ant which is effective but also could harm people who are susceptible to it; and guaiphenesin is a substance which is said to reduce the sticki-ness of sputum and thereby to help clear out blocked up sinuses. *Mu-Cron Liquid for Children* contains guaiphenesin and phenylpropanola-mine hydrochloride but no paracetamol and no ipecacuanha.

Dō-Dō Tablets contain ephedrine hydrochloride, caffeine, lobeline hydrochloride, theophylline sodium glycinate and salicylamide. Ephedrine hydrochloride is a similar substance to phenylpropanolamine hydrochloride and is equally harmful. Caffeine is, of course, a stimu-lant; it is discussed at greater length on p.174. Lobeline hydrochloride is a respiratory stimulant which has also been used as a smoking deter-rent with disappointing results (see p.159). Theophylline sodium glycinate is presumably included to help improve breathing; like lobeline hydrochloride it stimulates respiration. Salicylamide is a substance with properties similar to aspirin.

Both these products will work but under some circumstances the constituents can be dangerous. I do not recommend these tablets to anyone who has not first consulted a doctor. Both products have brief warnings on their packages.

Phenylephrine hydrochloride is present in a number of medicines designed to be taken orally. *Anapax Cold Tablets, Boots Cold Tablets with Vitamin C, Cold Discs, Coldrex Tablets, Esocol Cold Treatment Tablets* and *Lem-Sip* all contain it. Although its absorption from the gastrointestinal tract is rather unpredictable this powerful chemical can have an effect on the whole body – not just the nose or sinuses. It does not mix with a number of prescribed drugs, and it is potentially dangerous if taken by pregnant women or young children, or those with heart disease. As always, it is important to read and follow the manufacturer's instructions should you feel inclined to try any of these products.

Dristan Decongestant Tablets contain phenylephrine hydrochloride, together with aspirin and caffeine. *Cabdrivers Nasal Decongestant Tablets* contain paracetamol, salicylamide, caffeine and phenylephrine hydrochloride; *Penetrol Catarrh Lozenges* contain phenylephrine hydrochloride, too, while *Therex Decongestant Tablets* contain ephedrine sulphate and also atropine sulphate. *Bronchipax* tablets contain ephedrine resinate.

Many anti-catarrhal products seem to contain creosote, often in minute quantities. Creosote, which is perhaps best known as a wood preservative, has some properties as a disinfectant and an expectorant. It is present in the following products: *Boots Catarrh Cough Syrup (Creosoted), Boots Catarrh Pastilles, Famel Catarrh and Throat Pastilles, Heath and Heather's Catarrh Pastilles, Jackson's Bronchial Catarrh Pastilles, Potter's Catarrh Pastilles* and *Willocare Bronchial Catarrh Syrup*. Any one of these products may turn your urine green.

Then there are the nasal sprays and drops which contain drugs to relieve congestion. Again, these are often drugs such as phenylephrine which do indeed clear some of the congestion. Unhappily there is a snag about using these drugs directly on the nasal tissues. They can cause local irritation and when you stop using them you are quite likely to get the congestion back as bad as ever. To counteract this problem the obvious thing happens: people keep using their nasal spray. And that is damaging and dangerous.

Phenylephrine hydrochloride is a major constituent of *Anapax Nasal Spray, Biomydrin Nasal Spray, Coldrex Nasal Spray, Dristan Nasal Mist, Fenox Nasal Drops, Fenox Nasal Spray, Hayphryn Nasal Spray, Narex Nasal Spray, Nazex Nasal Spray, Neophryn Nasal Drops, Neophryn Nasal Spray, Snef Nasal Drops, Vibrocil Nasal Drops* and *Vibrocil Nasal Spray.*

Finally, there are the inhalants which contain aromatic oils and which can be very comforting. These are safe and effective and I do recommend them. You can either inhale them from hot water, sprinkle them on to a pillow or handkerchief or rub them on to your chest. Probably the best way of using an inhalant is to use it in hot water poured into a bowl and for this purpose non-branded inhalations are quite suitable. Try *Benzoin Inhalation BPC, Compound Benzoin Tincture BPC (Friar's Balsam), Menthol and Benzoin Inhalation BPC* or *Menthol Crystals*.

Many physicians suspect that it's the steam rather than the menthol which helps liquefy the secretions which are causing the congestion in the nose and sinuses but the drugs do at least make the whole business smell nice and medicinal.

Simply put hot water into a basin and add a few drops of one of the non-branded inhalants. Put a towel over your head and inhale the vapour for five minutes. That's all.

There are a number of commercially prepared inhalants available. Menthol is a major ingredient of *Boots Inhaler, Famel Inhalant Capsules, Famel Nasal Inhaler, Karvol Capsules, Medic-Aire Aerosol Cold Relief, Mentholatum Nasal Inhaler, Penetrol Inhalant, Three Flasks Handkerchief Inhalant, Vaderex Nasal Inhaler, Vapex Inhalant* and *Vicks Inhaler*.

Chest rubs, designed to be rubbed on to the chest and inhaled from there often contain menthol and camphor. The following products contain both these ingredients: *Boots Vapour Rub, Fisherman's Friend Rubbing Ointment, Fumic Vaporizing Rub, George's Vapour Rub, Rayglo Chest Rub, Vaderex Vapour Rub, Vapex Medicated Rub* and *Vicks Vapour Rub*.

Most of these useful substances contain other ingredients. Some contain antiseptics which are theoretically present to treat local infections but which are in practice likely to be quite ineffective. Many contain other pleasant smelling oils which have no real medicinal purpose.

Menthalin are handkerchiefs impregnated with a number of substances including menthol, and *Breathe Free Inhalant Tissues* are tissues impregnated with various oils. *Vicks Sinex Nasal Spray* contains oxymetazoline hydrochloride (a decongestant), menthol, camphor and eucalyptol.

The advantage of vapour rubs and inhalant capsules is that you can use them if you happen to be in circumstances where it is difficult to drape a towel over your head and obtain a basin full of hot water. A smear of *Vicks Vapour Rub* around your nose, or a *Karvol Capsule* broken on your handkerchief can prove handy.

Coughs

Coughing is a reflex response; it's a sign that your body is trying to eject an irritant. And basically it is a useful response. It can help get rid of a crumb of food or a bolus of phlegm stuck in your throat. So it is important to realize that if you are coughing it may be because your body knows best. If the cough isn't painful, doesn't keep you awake for hours at a time and does produce sputum, then you'd be wise to avoid treating it. It's worth remembering that more people die because they *can't* cough than die because they *do* cough.

When a cough doesn't bring up any sputum, when it is associated with pain, or when it keeps you from resting then it might be worth doing something about; particularly if it lasts for more than a few days without improving.

There are several things you can do to ease a cough *without* buying medicine. Most importantly you can stop smoking or keep out of the way of people who do smoke. Children who suffer a lot from coughs very often have at least one parent who smokes regularly. You don't have to be a smoker to suffer from the effects of cigarette smoke.

Avoid sudden changes in temperature and keep the rooms in which you sit warm and well ventilated. Hot drinks, such as *Peggy Coleman's Hot Lemon Drink* (see p.85), may help any cough, and a steam inhalation (see p.77) may prove restful and productive. During the daytime, sucking a boiled sweet or lozenge may help; the sweet doesn't have to be medicated. Many of the so-called 'cough sweets' are little more than ordinary sweets at extraordinary prices.

Cough medicines

There are two types of cough medicine: suppressants and expectorants.

Suppressants are supposed to simply suppress the cough reflex. Codeine, pholcodeine, morphine noscapine and dextrorphan are common ingredients in suppressant cough medicines (a large proportion of the world's narcotic supply is used in cough remedies).

Expectorants are supposed to liquefy and loosen phlegm and help you cough it up. Acetic acid, ammonium salts, creosote, ipecacuanha, liquorice, garlic, guaiphenesin, gumweed, soapwort, squill and tolu are common ingredients of expectorant cough medicines.

Many branded cough medicines contain both an expectorant and a suppressant, usually in very small quantities. You may think that there is something rather illogical about including both types of ingredient. You'd have the support of a number of pharmacologists. Together with these main substances many manufacturers also include other drugs such as aniseed, menthol and peppermint. Antihistamines are often included but I'm not sure why. A number of medicines include substances designed to relieve wheezing and dilate the air passages within the lungs. I don't recommend these products at all – they can be dangerous for those who are susceptible to them. If you have difficulty in breathing or find yourself wheezing then you need to see a doctor.

The simplest, cheapest, safest and probably most effective suppressant cough linctuses are *Pholcodine Linctus BPC* and *Opiate Squill Linctus BPC* (*Gee's Linctus*), but a steam inhalation (see p.77) may prove more helpful, and indeed inhalations are the most effective and economical expectorants.

Sucking sweets can help relieve a cough in several ways. Firstly, the increase in saliva will ensure that the back of the mouth and the throat are kept moist. Secondly, any soothing substance in the sweet (honey, glycerin, liquorice, camphor, menthol, chloroform, peppermint, eucalyptus, cinnamon, lemon and so on) will help the same areas.

Sweets are better than linctuses or mixtures for the simple reason that they are sucked for several minutes at a time. A linctus only has as long as it takes to go down your throat to soothe.

There are literally scores and scores of different branded cough medicines on the market. As examples I have listed here the contents of some of the best-selling remedies – all of these, incidentally, are commonly prescribed by doctors as well as being available without a prescription. *Actifed Compound Linctus* contains triprolidine hydrochloride (an antihistamine), pseudoephedrine hydrochloride (a decongestant) and codeine phosphate (a cough suppressant). *Benylin Expectorant* is probably the biggest-selling cough medicine in Britain. It contains diphenhydramine hydrochloride (an antihistamine), ammonium chloride, sodium citrate and menthol. *Dimotane Expectorant* contains brompheniramine maleate (the apparently obligatory antihistamine), guaiphenesin (an expectorant), phenylephrine hydrochloride and phenylpropanolamine hydrochloride (decongestants). *Linctified* contains triprolidine hydrochloride (an antihistamine), pseudoephedrine hydrochloride, codeine phosphate and guaiphenesin (an expectorant). *Phensedyl* contains promethazine hydrochloride (an antihistamine), codeine phosphate and ephedrine hydrochloride (a decongestant). *Tixylix* contains promethazine hydrochloride, pholcodine (a cough suppressant) and phenylpropanolamine hydrochloride.

Many patent cough remedies contain a large number of different ingredients. Inevitably each substance is present only in a minute quantity and I believe that these linctuses and mixtures are really not worth considering.

I have composed a list of cough medicines which contain small amounts of five or more ingredients. Here it is: *Adult Cough Balsam, Anapax Triple Action Cough Mixture, Ayrtons Bronchial Emulsion (Extra Strong), Barkoff Cough Syrup, Boots Children's Cough Linctus, Bronal Cough and Catarrh Elixir, Brontussin, Buttercup Syrup, Cabdrivers Adult Linctus, Carters Vegetable Cough Remover, Castellan Cough Syrup for Children, Castellan No. 10 Cough Mixture, Congreve's Valsamic Elixir, Cox's Antitussive Linctus, Cox's Bronchial Balsam, Cox's Catarrh and Bronchial Syrup, Cox's Children's Cherry Cough Syrup, Cox's Extra Strong Bronchial Mixture, Curraglen Bronchial Mixture, Deakin's Cough and Cold Healer, Duttons Cough Mixture, Eldermint Cough Mixture, Extra Strong Bronchial Mixture, Fisherman's Friend Family Cough Linctus, Hactos Chest and Cough Mixture, Heath and Heather's Balm of Gilead Cough Mixture, Hills Bronchial Balsam, Hills Junior Balsam, Honey Kof Syrup, Junior Kil Kof, Kil Kof, Lanes Honey and Molasses Cough Mixture, Lem-Eze Cough Linctus, Lem-Mel Chest and Lung Syrup, Liqufruta with Honey, Liqufruta Lemon, Liqufruta Medica, Liqufruta Standard, Mayfair A Mentholated*

Balsam, Meltus Adult Cough and Catarrh Linctus, Meltus Junior Cough and Catarrh Linctus, Mentholated Bronchial Balsam, Nurse Sykes Bronchial Balsam, Owbridges Cough Mixture, Parkinsons Glycerine Lemon, Potter's Balm of Gilead Cough Mixture, Potter's Vegetable Cough Remover, Robert's Croupline Cough Syrup, Savory and Moore Cherry Cough Linctus, Savory and Moore Mentholated Balsam, Savory and Moore Terperoin Elixir, Sure Shield Rum Cough Elixir, Three Flasks Blackcurrant Cough Linctus, Three Flasks Bronchial Emulsion, Three Flasks Children's Cherry Flavoured Cough Syrup, Three Noughts Cough Syrup, Tusana Sedative Linctus, Vicks Expectorant Cough Syrup, Willocare Adults Bronchial Balsam and *Zubes Cough Mixture*.

Just as there are a number of cough linctuses and mixtures which contain five or more ingredients in minute quantities, so there are a number of cough pastilles which contain a similar mixture of medicinal substances. Here are some of them: *Boots Bronchial Lozenges, Hacks, Heath and Heather's Balm of Gilead Cough Pastilles, Hills Bronchial Balsam Pastilles, Liqufruta Cough Pastilles, Meditus Pastilles* and *Wigglesworth Adults Bronchial Balsam Pastilles*.

I do not recommend any of these medicinal cocktails.

Warning Since many cough medicines contain a good deal of alcohol it is possible to become quite drunk when you think you're just trying to get rid of a cough if you exceed the recommended dose. It is important to remember this if you drive and take cough medicines. The antihistamines included in cough medicines may cause drowsiness and are therefore also dangerous for drivers (see p.39).

Sore throats
There are many causes of sore throats. The overdry air of a centrally-heated building, the continued inhalation of cigarette smoke and talking for hours at a time are just three causes. A cold, a blocked nose and a straightforward infection of the throat are three more.

Most sore throats can be cleared without penicillin. Keep quiet if you can, avoid cigarette smoke, have plenty of hot drinks and to clear out your mouth (if it feels like the proverbial parrot's cage floor) gargle with half a teaspoonful of salt in a glass of warm water. That's just as good as any branded gargle you can buy. Take aspirin or paracetamol (see p. 134) for the pain and suck any sweet you fancy to increase the flow of saliva, thereby keeping your throat moist and therefore less painful. Peppermints are probably better than boiled sweets and they aren't as bad for your teeth. Antiseptic lozenges are a waste of money since they can't possibly eradicate all the germs in your throat. They won't be any more soothing than any other sort of sweet.

Many lozenges, pastilles and sweets sold for the relief of sore throats contain antiseptics. Antiseptics are ingredients in the following products: *Biothrin Lozenges, Boots Antiseptic Lozenges, Boots Iodized Throat Tablets, De Witt's Throat Lozenges, Dequadin, Evans Antiseptic Throat Pastilles, Jackson's Antiseptic Throat Pastilles, Jackson's Sore Throat Lozenges, Labosept, Merocets, Mentholatum Antiseptic Lozenges, Simpkins Sore Throat Antiseptic Mini Tabs, Sterling Health Antiseptic Throat Lozenges, Strepsils, Sure Shield Antibiotic Throat Lozenges, Sure Shield Iodized Throat Lozenges, TCP Throat Pastilles, Tetrazets, Tyrocane Throat Lozenges, Tyroco Throat Lozenges, Tyrosolven* and *Tyrozets.*

Since several of the products sold as aids for colds and sore throats are made by confectioners rhather than drug companies it is not surprising that a number of pastilles and sweets sold for sore throats are extremely mild – being nothing much more than sweets in fact. To select the best buy judge by the size of the packet, the price and the taste!

Apart from antiseptic lozenges sore throats can be tackled with antiseptics in other ways. *TCP Liquid Antiseptic* is recommended by its manufacturers for the relief of a sore throat, as is *Betadine Gargle and Mouthwash.* But as I have said, an ordinary salt gargle (half a teaspoonful in a glass of warm water) may be just as effective and soothing. Gargling with a solution made out of soluble aspirin helps. *Aspergum* is a chewable form of aspirin which is useful in the treatment of sore throats when gargling is not practicable.

Multipurpose cold remedies

In recent years a number of products have been successfully promoted as multipurpose remedies designed to ease various symptoms of the common cold.

Night Nurse contains promethazine hydrochloride (an antihistamine which can cause drowsiness), pholcodine (a cough suppressant which can cause drowsiness), paracetamol and alcohol. *Vicks MediNite* contains ephedrine sulphate (a drug which when given in adequate dosage can prevent wheezing), doxylamine succinate (an antihistamine type of drug that causes drowsiness), dextromethorphan hydrobromide (a cough suppressant similar to pholcodine but which does not cause drowsiness), paracetamol and alcohol. The drowsiness caused by the constituents is in this case likely to be an advantage.

A number of big-selling drugs are based on the ubiquitous lemon. For example, *Lem-Sip* contains paracetamol, phenylephrine hydrochloride (a popular decongestant), sodium citrate (which has a mild value as a laxative and diuretic) and vitamin C. *Lemonexa* contains codeine phosphate (a cough suppressant), ephedrine hydrochloride (a decongestant) and diphenhydramine hydrochloride (an antihistamine).

Contac 400 are sustained release capsules which contain phenylpropanolamine hydrochloride (a decongestant) and hyoscyamine sulphate (which can reduce secretions). *10 Hour Capsules* contain paracetamol, noscapine (a cough suppressant similar to pholcodine), terpin hydrate (which increases bronchial secretions) and phenylephrine hydrochloride. *10 Hour Fever Cold Mixture* contains quinine hydrochloride, totaquine and quinine sulphate (all mild analgesics and antipyretics), also nitric acid, hydrochloric acid and eucalyptus oil. *Clear Night Tablets* contain pholcodine and promethazine hydrochloride.

In my view none of these products are worth buying, but if you do try them, follow the manufacturer's instructions.

Aspirin (see p.134) is a major ingredient of many cold remedies. *Beechams Powders* (available in powder or tablet form), for example, are primarily a mixture of aspirin and caffeine. Two aspirin tablets and a cup of coffee might be cheaper.

Paracetamol is present in useful quantities in *Anapax Cold Tablets, Boots Cold Relief Tablets, Boots Cold Tablets, Cold Discs, Coldrex Powders, Coldrex Tablets* and *Esocol Cold Treatment Tablets. Coldrex Tablets, Anapax* and *Boots Cold Tablets* also contain caffeine, while all except *Boots Cold Relief Sachets* also contain phenylephrine hydrochloride (see p.76).

The following products for coughs, colds, sore throats, catarrh and flu have not yet been mentioned here. Some of them are advertised by their manufacturers as suitable for a number of different symptoms and some are simply expensive versions of easily obtainable remedies. None of these products seem to me to be worth discussing individually and I doubt if the disappearance of all of them would have any effect on the health of the nation.

Anapax Adult's Cough Linctus, Antifect, Ayrtons Children's Cough Syrup, Boots Children's Cough Pastilles, Boots Glycerin, Honey and Lemon Linctus (with or without ipecacuanha), *Boots Glycerin of Thymol Pastilles, Boots Lozenges of Linseed, Boots Menthol and Eucalyptol Pastilles, Boots Menthol and Eucalyptus Throat Drops, Boots Old-Fashioned Cough Drops, Bron-Skels Pastilles, Campbell's Cherry Flavoured Cough Syrup, CB Coltsfoot Bronchials, Children's Cherry Cough Linctus, Cough and Sore Throat Pastilles, Covonia Mentholated Bronchial Balsam, Creds, Deakin's Fever and Inflammation Remedy, Doctor's Catarrh Pastilles, Evans Bronchial Cough Mixture, Famel Honey and Lemon Cough Linctus, Family Cherry Linctus, Fennings' Original Mixture Folk Pastilles, Fisherman's Friend Throat and Chest Lozenges, Galloway's Baby Cough Linctus, Galloway's Bronchial Expectorant, Galloway's Cough Syrup, Galloway's Lung Syrup, Garlic Plus Remedy, Garlodex, Geeps Pastilles, Halls Cherry Flavoured Cough Drops, Jackson's Eucalyptus and Menthol Pastilles, Jackson's Bronchial Lozenges, Jackson's Febrifuge, Jackson's Glycerin Thymol Pastilles, Jackson's Linseed, Liquorice and Chlorodyne Lozenges, Jackson's Mentholated Bronchial Pastilles, Jackson's Night Cough Pastilles, Jackson's Pholcodine Pastilles, Keybells Glycerin and Honey with Lemon, Keybells Glycerin, Lemon and Ipecac, Lemon Flu-Cold Syrup, Mac Lozenges, Mac Lozenges Honey Lem, Meggezones, Mentho Lyptus Blackcurrant, Mentho Lyptus Extra Strong, Mentho Lyptus Honey and Lemon, Mentho Lyptus Liquorice and Aniseed, Mentho Lyptus Original, Mentho Lyptus Raspberry and Honey, Premier Bronchial Pastilles, Pulmo Bailly, Respaton Lozenges, Ress-Q Pastilles, Sandersons Cough Linctus, Sandersons Throat Specific Mixture, Sandersons Throat Specific Pastilles, Simpkins Bronchial Drops, Simpkins Brown Treacle Cough Drops, Simpkins Catarrh Mini Tabs, Simpkins Children's Cough Drops, Simpkins Menthol and Eucalyptus Drops, Simpkins Menthol and Eucalyptus Mini Tabs, Simpkins Sulphur Drops, Simpkins TCL Drops, Simpkins Teddy Cough Mini Tabs, Tusana Cough Pastilles, Tusana Sedative Linctus, Tusana Cough Lozenges, Tussobron Pastilles, Tussobron Cough Suppressant Syrup, Valda Pastilles, Veno's Cough Mixture, Veno's Honey and Lemon Cough Mixture, Vicks Formula 44 Antihistamine Antitussive Expectorant Cough Mixture, Vicks Formula 44 Cough Discs, Vicks Lozenges Blackcurrant Flavour, Vicks Lozenges Lemon with Vitamin C, Vicks Lozenges Regular Menthol, Vicks*

Lozenges Wild Cherry, Wigglesworth Compound Syrup of Honey, Glycerin and Blackcurrant, Willocare Bronchial Mixture and *Willocare Mentholated Balsam.*

Many readers will recognize personal favourites on this list of remedies. Faith is a powerful influence in the effectiveness of any medicine and if you feel particularly enthusiastic about a product then it will very probably have a greater effect than might be expected.

Finally a word about the Fennings' products which are so popular that it is perhaps worthwhile examining them individually.

Fennings' Adult Cooling Powders contain caffeine (a stimulant), paracetamol (a painkiller), magnesium carbonate (an antacid) and kaolin (usually used to help clear up diarrhoea).

Fennings' Children's Cooling Powders contain paracetamol.

Fennings' Little Healers contain ipecacuanha (to help a cough).

Fennings' Mixture, Lemon Flavoured contains a close relative of aspirin, oil of lemon and a little chloroform.

Fennings' Original Mixture contains nitric acid (which in larger quantities has been used to remove warts) and peppermint oil (which hasn't).

Fennings' Soluble Children's Cooling Tablets contain paracetamol, sodium bicarbonate (often used as an antacid) and magnesium carbonate (an antacid).

Fennings' Soluble Junior Aspirin contains aspirin.

Peggy Coleman's Hot Lemon Drink

My wife has a marvellous recipe for producing a lemon drink which helps relieve most of the symptoms of a cold. She tells me that you slice five lemons into two pints of cold water and add two tablespoonfuls of sugar or honey. Bring it all to the boil and simmer, reducing the liquid slightly. Then allow to cool. Afterwards you can keep the concentrate and add hot water to it as you like. If you serve it in a large glass and sniff the rising fumes you can use the drink as an inhalant and a soothing remedy for an irritated throat.

It will do you just as much good as any bottle from the chemist's shop, and it can't do you any harm.

When to see a doctor

Unless you cough up blood or discoloured sputum, suffer chest pains or become exceptionally breathless you can leave a cough for ten days before seeking medical advice.

After a cold or attack of flu pains across the front of your head and stuffiness which suggest catarrh can be treated at home for ten days.

A sore throat doesn't need to be left so long. Give it five days and then go and see your family doctor who may feel that the time has come to introduce an antibiotic into your life.

CONSTIPATION

Before discussing the home medicines available for the treatment of constipation the symptom undoubtedly needs to be defined. For it is an indisputable paradox that one man's constipation can be another's diarrhoea.

Some people consider that they are constipated if they do not have their bowels opened at least three times a day, producing a complete and satisfying result on each occasion. Others, more accustomed to gentler activity, will only complain if their once a week routine is disturbed. Those who would like to compare their own bowel habits with the statistical norm might be interested to know that over half of the general population have their bowels open only once a day – most commonly just after breakfast. The majority of the population perform between three times a day and three times a week but there are many whose habits fall outside these purely arbitrary borders.

Clearly, therefore, it is not possible to produce any precise definition of constipation. All that can be said is that if an individual's bowels are appreciably more sluggish than is normal for him or for her then he or she is constipated!

Inevitably, it's the type of food that is eaten that is most frequently responsible for the development of a constipated bowel. It is, after all, perfectly logical that what is eaten should have a vital influence over what is excreted. Too many cakes, chocolates, sweets and puddings will slow things up, as will too much strong tea, I'm afraid.

Similarly most bouts of constipation can be successfully reversed by a carefully organized dietary programme. It's helpful to eat plenty of fresh fruit (oranges are particularly good), green vegetables and salads. And it's useful to·drink plenty of fluids – particularly fruit juices. Wholemeal cereals may also help to keep things moving. It should already be clear that the vast majority of people who take laxatives do not need them. Many simply have bowels which need to be emptied less frequently than their owners consider seemly. And many more, who have acquired sluggish bowels, could solve their problems permanently, easily and safely merely by changing their dietary intake.

The only genuine indication for the use of a laxative is a persistent change in the frequency with which the bowels are emptied which cannot be explained or rectified by a dietary change and which is not accompanied by any other unexplained symptom such as pain, intermittent diarrhoea or the passing of blood.

It is sometimes necessary to use laxatives after an operation, after childbirth or during some long-term illness which necessitates bedrest and makes normal activities impossible. It may be wise to use a laxative when the addition of fresh fruit, wholewheat cereals, bran and plenty of fluids has not solved a persistent and perhaps even uncomfortable problem. But it should never be forgotten that the unwise over-enthusiastic use of 'opening' medicines can cause bowel damage, sometimes with the result that laxatives become a long-term necessity.

Bulk-forming laxatives
Laxatives in this group work in a natural way to stimulate the bowel and I therefore recommend them. Foods such as wholemeal cereals and fruits give the muscles of the bowel something to get to grips with, thereby encouraging muscular activity and resultant bowel emptying. The bulk-forming laxatives work in the same way.

When available as granules or tablets they need to be taken with plenty of water; they swell inside the bowel and work within twelve to twenty-four hours. However, cereals such as *All Bran, Weetabix* and *Shredded Wheat,* muesli such as *Alpen,* and bran tablets work in precisely the same way and can be just as safe and effective.

Medicinal laxatives designed to work in this way usually contain bran, methylcellulose, psyllium, agar, sterculia or ispaghula husk. *Scotts Husky Wholemeal and Bran Biscuits* contain bran; *Fybogel, Isogel* and *Vi-Siblin* are preparations of ispaghula husk; *Blandlax* contains a cellulose product (together with magnesium hydroxide); *Celevac* contains methylcellulose, as do *Cellucon* and *Cologel*; and *Normacol* contains sterculia. Psyllium is a major ingredient of *Metamucil,* and *Innerfresh* contains agar. These products are all safe and effective.

Lubricants

Lubricants, which assist the passage of faeces by easing the way and softening the stools are fattening since they consist of oils which may be digested. Lubricant laxatives are particularly useful for painful anorectal disorders since they produce a smooth and easily passed stool and patients with anal fissures or piles may find them particularly helpful. Some, however, may find the occasional leakage of fluid from the back passage annoying and embarrassing.

Liquid paraffin, which is available under several brand names, works well but it is messy and may interfere with the absorption of vitamins A, D and K – all of which are fat-soluble vitamins. Liquid paraffin is sold as *Liquid Paraffin Emulsion BP* and is also available in mixture with other substances. It is, for example, available together with magnesium hydroxide as *Cremaffin* and as *Mil-Par*.

Well-known products such as *Dulcodos* (which also contains bisacodyl) contain lubricant materials. Dioctyl sodium sulphosuccinate, which is present in both *Dulcodos* and *Normax,* is also used to soften ear wax and as a spermicide.

Stimulants

Stimulants or irritants, which act directly on the bowel wall and urge it into activity, can be dangerous and should be used very carefully. They may cause griping pains.

The biggest-selling product in this group is undoubtedly *Senokot*. *Senokot* consists of senna, as do a number of other products, including *Bidrolar, Boots Senna Laxative Tablets, Heatherclean, Heatherlax Constipation Tablets, Pru-Sen* and another big-selling product, *California Syrup of Figs.* It is important to note that products such as *Potter's Lion Cleansing Herbs* which are advertised as being purely 'herbal' and which are said to 'contain no drugs whatsoever' do, in fact, contain senna leaf. The advertising material for *Potter's Lion Cleansing Herbs* claims that senna leaf is 'probably the simplest and most harmless natural laxative'. Senna is, in fact, a fairly powerful stimulant purgative.

Cascara, rhubarb and aloes have similar action to products based on senna. Bisacodyl, a member of the same group as senna and cascara, is best known as *Dulcolax* or *Dulcodos*. They all work in about six to twelve hours and should be taken the night before for a result the morning after. *Dulcolax Suppositories* act in twenty to sixty minutes.

Castor oil, which is sold as *Castor Oil BP*, is a time-honoured stimulant laxative which works in two to six hours. It should be given on an empty stomach since it has to be digested before it can work. It acts on the small intestine and has a very dramatic effect in even modest doses. There is not much point in taking more than 20–30 ml. If given to a pregnant woman it may start off a premature labour so its use should obviously be avoided in these circumstances.

Another well-used stimulant is phenolphthalein for which, according to *Drugs of Choice 1978–79*, 'there are no medical indications'. This extremely well-established substance is one of the most commonly used ingredients in laxatives sold for use at home. The following products include phenolphthalein: *Agarol, Boldolaxine, Bonomint Laxative Chewing Gum, Brooklax Chocolate Laxative, Carter's Little Liver Pills, Delax, Ex-Lax Junior, Ex-Lax Pills, Ex-Lax Tablets, Fam-Lax Laxative Tablets, Feen-a-mint, Juno Junipah Tablets, Kest, Nylax* (described in advertisements as 'the gentle vitamin and herbal laxative'), *Peplax, Reg-u-letts* and *Sure Shield Laxatives*.

Generally speaking, stimulant laxatives should be kept for emergencies and *never* used repeatedly. People whose bowels are 'addicted' to stimulants are the exception to this rule.

Salts

Salts keep water in the bowel. They tend to be rather drastic since they work very quickly and can produce watery diarrhoea within an hour or two, and they need to be used with extreme caution. The main danger of using salts as purgatives is that they can produce an imbalance of salts in the body. Compounds containing sodium sulphate (such as *Juno Junipah Salts*) are among the fastest acting. Magnesium hydroxide (*Milk of Magnesia*) is one of the mildest of the saline cathartics. It is also one of the top-selling laxative products as is

Andrews Liver Salt – a combination of citric acid, sodium bicarbonate, magnesium sulphate and sucrose. Other health salts such as *Eno Fruit Salt, Epsom Salts (Magnesium Sulphate BP)*, and *Glauber Salts (Sodium Sulphate BP)* have a laxative action.

Lactulose

Available most commonly as *Duphalac* this remedy is mild, natural, slow and rather expensive. It consists of a sugar which cannot be used like other sugars in our bodies but which is passed through into the large bowel. There it provides small bacteria with a feast and is broken down into acids which stimulate bowel movement. The usual initial dose is 10–20 g and lactulose may take two to three days to work. In high dosage it may cause nausea, diarrhoea and wind.

Mixed blessings

There are a number of laxatives on sale which contain several different constituents. Among the most exotic mixtures are *Beechams Pills* which contain ginger, coriander, hard soap, aloes, rosemary oil, juniper oil, anise oil, capsicum oleoresin, ginger oleoresin and light magnesium carbonate; *Bile Beans* which contain cascara, jalap, peppermint oil and ginger, capsicum oleoresin, colocynth, aloes, cardamom fruit, ipomoea resin, sodium tauroglycocholate, powdered gentian and liquorice; *Boldo Tablets* which contain cascara, fucus, uva ursi extract and boldo extract; *Brandreth's Pills* which contain cascara, aloes, guaiacum resin, capsicum and hard soap; *George's Special Pills for Chronic Constipation* which contain podophyllum resin, ginger, gambogex, jalap, colocynth, aloes, curd soap and caraway oil and *Pylatum Regulators* which consist of a mixture of senna, cascara, aloin, colocynth, ginger oleoresin, peppermint oil and hard soap.

Many of these 'mixed blessings' contain small amounts of very powerful laxatives. Jalap and podophyllum, for example, are drastic purgatives which may cause severe irritation to the bowel if used in large quantities. These substances have been largely replaced by other laxatives on their own but still appear in mixtures.

Traditional *Syrup of Figs* consists of figs, rhubarb, senna, cascara and sucrose.

Suppositories

There is a great deal of support behind the use of suppositories in France and other European countries across the Channel. In Britain suppositories are still considered rather nasty and distasteful by most people. Some even complain that it is impossible to expect a medicine to work if you push it into your anus. Laxatives given by suppository are, however, effective and quick to work. Glycerin suppositories which act simply by dissolving and easing the way for hard stools are gentlest. *Dulcolax* is also available in this form.

Enemas

Enemas (see p.46) can be allowed to run into the bowel by gravity, or they can be pumped into place. They may be given entirely for their laxative effect or for other medicinal purposes. Many varieties of enema are available. These remedies are, however, best prescribed and used by experts.

Conclusion

If you take regular doses of laxatives you're likely to suffer from colic, wind and watery diarrhoea. As your bowels become insensitive to normal demands and require stimulating more and more often, so laxatives may induce chronic constipation. They should, therefore, be used with great care.

If you feel that you are suffering from constipation try adjusting your diet before resorting to medicinal compounds. If that fails then I suggest a bulk-forming laxative as the most natural way to stimulate bowel activity. If you have some other favourite use that.

And if then, after five days, your constipation has not resolved visit your doctor for advice. Do not persist for more than five days with any laxative medicine.

CONTRACEPTION

There was a time when contraceptives were kept well out of sight in chemists' shops. For a man, purchasing a supply of condoms meant either struggling to tell a shy young girl what was required in a series of broad hints or else braving a disapproving look from a matron who could not have been more threatening had she been the mother of his intended. I don't know what it was like for a woman. But it can't have been much better.

Today, that has all changed. In most chemists' shops contraceptives are lined up at the front of the counter, sharing pride of place with the aspirin tablets, gripe water and vitamin pills.

Two main types of contraceptives can be bought without medical advice and have real value in pregnancy avoidance.

Firstly, there are condoms (also known as sheaths, French letters, rubber johnnies and *Durex*) which are used regularly by about one quarter of the couples requiring contraception. Only in recent years has the pill edged ahead of the sheath in popularity and as women in their thirties are taken off the pill the chances are that the sheath will once again move back into first place. Used properly this is an extremely effective form of contraception. One survey showed that if a hundred couples used the sheath for one year, only three or four women would become pregnant.

Secondly, there are the spermicides, chemicals which literally kill off the sperm and thereby prevent conception. Spermicides are used far less widely as a sole means of contraception as some doctors believe that they are not completely reliable.

Other contraceptives which may be bought over the counter are not worth considering. Douches, for example, which are favoured by some women can just as easily wash sperms up into the womb as wash them out of the vagina.

Condoms

This form of contraception used to be compared to 'paddling with wellingtons on' or 'playing the piano with gloves on' because of the fact that with a thick layer of rubber separating the penis from the vagina the joys of sex were rather slight. Today's disposable contraceptives are usually thin enough to ensure that the loss of sensation is slight.

The advantages of using condoms are presumably fairly obvious; they're useful for unpremeditated sexual encounters; they're available for use by everyone regardless of medical history or condition; they provide some protection against venereal disease; and they're easy to get hold of. Even if you can't find a chemist's shop open the gentlemen's lavatory in the nearest public house will probably be equipped with an automatic dispensing machine (upon which there will undoubtedly be scribbled slogans like 'buy me and stop one' and 'this chewing gum tastes awful').

The disadvantages are that using them embarrasses some people and diminishes sensation for others. (Diminishing sensation helps some men who are premature ejaculators. The thin layer of rubber twixt penis and vagina helps ensure that the erection lasts longer.) They occasionally fail. To keep the risks of becoming pregnant to a minimum it is important to follow certain basic rules when using a condom.

1 A condom should always be put on as soon as the penis is erect. Sperm can leak out of the penis before ejaculation.
2 Any air at the end of the condom should be expelled as it is rolled on to the penis. If the air is allowed to remain the condom is more likely to burst (although modern condoms are so strong that you really can blow them up into balloons). If the condom does not have a teat make sure that there is some space left at the end.
3 Handle condoms with care. Sharp nails and teeth can burst them.
4 After ejaculation the penis should be removed from the vagina with the condom still in place. One partner should simply hold on to the rim of the sheath and make sure that it doesn't slip off.

Choosing a condom
Condoms are available in many different shapes and colours these days. The only thing that doesn't really vary is size – condoms will stretch to fit even the largest organ. You can buy condoms that are straight or contoured, dry or lubricated, smooth or rippled, transparent or coloured and thin or very thin. You can buy them with or without teats at the end to hold the sperm and you can, if you're willing to forgo sensitivity for the sake of economy, buy very thick, washable condoms.

The most important single thing to look for when choosing a condom is the British Standards kitemark which confirms that the product (or more accurately ones like it) has been tested and found to be safe and reliable. Apart from that it's largely a matter of taste, although most experts agree that the very short 'American tips' which leave the shaft of the penis uncovered are *not* safe – they tend to come off too easily – and the particularly fancy condoms which are fitted with lots of knobs and projections designed to stimulate a woman are not safe because they may rip or burst.

The thickness of condoms is measured in thousandths of a millimetre and most sheaths fall into one of two groups. The thicker (and usually the cheaper) are 0.065 mm thick. This group includes *Atlas* (lubricated with a teat), ordinary *Durex* (non-lubricated and available with or without a teat), *Durex Allergy* (non-lubricated without a teat and designed to minimize the chances of either partner developing signs of an allergic reaction as a result of contact with the sheath – if this condom doesn't prove adequately non-allergic, non-synthetic sheaths are available which are made from sheep's intestines), *Durex Gossamer* (lubricated and available with or without a teat), *Durex Nu-form* (designed to accommodate the shape of the penis, lubricated and with a teat), *Durex Unison* (which is ribbed for extra stimulation), *Forget-me-not* (lubricated with a teat) and *Two's Company* (lubricated, with a teat and available in a pack with a spermicidal pessary).

The thinner (and more expensive) group are made of rubber which is 0.05 mm thick. Brands in this group include *Durex Black Shadow* (made in black), *Durex Fetherlite* and *Durex Fiesta* (available in a variety of pretty colours). All these sheaths are lubricated.

In addition to these varieties there is a sheath called *Durex Nu-Form 'Extra Safe'* which has its own spermicidal lubricant. The purpose of the lubricant is, naturally, to aid penetration. A dry rubber sheath may prove uncomfortable. Making the lubricant spermicidal simply adds to the effectiveness of the protection provided. In the next section I shall discuss spermicides.

Spermicides

The first thing to be said about spermicides is that they should not be used without some form of mechanical protection. Spermicides may be designed to kill sperms but they are not by any means guaranteed to kill all sperms. A man with a high sperm count may have plenty left even after the spermicidal cream has killed off many millions of sperm.

So don't use any spermicide by itself.

Spermicides are available as creams, pessaries, aerosol foams, gels, foaming tablets and impregnated soluble films. They should be put into the vagina a few minutes before intercourse (enough to allow time for them to spread around but not enough to allow time for them to leak out) and replaced at hourly intervals if intercourse is prolonged or repeated.

One of the best-known spermicides available today is *C Film*, a small square of spermicide-impregnated film which, it is said, can be placed either inside the vagina or on top of the penis. According to the *Handbook of Contraceptive Practice* published by the Department of Health and Social Security this product 'is relatively ineffective and should not be advised'. So I won't.

Apart from the fact that they are messy, that they taste nasty and that they are not very effective there isn't anything wrong with spermicides. They should keep for about a year, but keep them in the refrigerator if the weather is hot and keep an eye on the expiry dates. If you keep pessaries in the fridge do make sure that no one makes a jelly or decorates a cake with them. It has happened.

Choosing a spermicide

Most spermicides contain a chemical called nonoxynol 9. Varieties containing this substance include *C Film, Delfen Cream, Delfen Foam, Duracreme, Duragel, Ortho-Creme, Rendell's Pessaries, Staycept Pessaries* and *Two's Company Pessaries*. Nonoxynol 9 is mixed with benzethonium chloride in *Emko* foaming aerosol and *Orthoforms* pessaries. Other products, which include such sensual-sounding chemicals as p-di-isobutylphenoxypolyethoxyethanol and tri-isopropylphenoxypole-thoxyethanol are *Antemin Cream, Genexol Pessaries, Ortho-gynol Jelly, Preceptin Jelly* and *Staycept Jelly*.

CRAMPS

When people talk about getting cramp, they usually mean in their legs. In fact, although these painful, spasmodic contractions can attack muscles anywhere, it is usually the muscles at the back of the legs which are involved. Poor, overstretched or interrupted circulation is usually the cause, and, rarely, excessive sweating, which produces salt depletion, can also cause cramps.

Older people often get cramps at night and to prevent these they may be tempted to buy one or other of the proprietary preparations which are available.

Crampex Tablets contain guaiphenesin, nicotinic acid, calcium gluconate and calciferol. *Limb-Ease Tablets* contain a modest dose of a vasodilator designed to increase the flow of blood to the muscles. These products may help.

Old wives' remedies include putting a cork under the pillow, putting brimstone under your mattress or carrying a mole's foot in your pocket. For cramp in the legs a mole's hindfoot is said to be most efficacious. No research seems to have been done on this point.

There is a useful exercise which can be tried if you suffer badly from night cramps in your legs.

Three times a day stand facing a wall two or three feet away from you. (You need to be barefoot for this exercise by the way.) Lean forward keeping your heels on the floor and touch the wall with your hands. You'll feel your calf muscles tightening as you do this. Hold the position for ten seconds, rest, and then do it again. If you do this three times a day for a week and then repeat it occasionally once a day or after heavy exercise you may find that the night cramps no longer bother you.

CUTS, SCRATCHES, GRAZES, BRUISES, BURNS, SCALDS AND ABRASIONS

Antiseptics and germicides are stocked in two out of three homes: *Germolene* and *Savlon* being two of the most commonly bought products. Some people seem to feel that they are behaving irresponsibly if they do not smother any minor abrasion with an antiseptic cream or douse any injured area with disinfectant. In fact there is very little point in using these products other than to make 'nurse' and 'patient' feel that something useful has been done.

The human body is really very good at arranging its own repairs when minor damage has been done (I am assuming that medical advice will be sought for major wounds). When you cut yourself the blood you lose helps wash dirt and germs away from the wound. Within a few minutes the blood in the wound will clot and form a hard protective scab; any dirt and debris left inside the scab will be cleared up by scavenging white blood cells. The hard scab will remain in place, as a protective shield, until the skin underneath has been repaired.

All this goes on without any outside interference. The body's natural defence mechanisms work more effectively when the wound is left exposed to the air. If occlusive dressings are put over small wounds the skin becomes soft and soggy and is more likely to harbour infection. Antiseptic ointments and creams are unlikely to help speed up healing and they may actually interfere with and delay natural protective processes.

Cleaning a wound

Antiseptics and disinfectants are substances that either destroy micro-organisms or inhibit their growth. Ordinary substances available for home use will kill off a small proportion of the organisms which have permanently or temporarily taken up residence on the skin but they will leave many more alive and well. It is the body's own defence mechanisms which provide the most effective protection.

The best way that you can help your body is simply to wash any damaged skin with clean, running cold water. If you scrub at the wound gently you will remove dirt, hair, superficial bacteria and dead skin and prepare the area for natural healing. Removing dirt is the most important thing you can do to speed up natural healing. Once the affected area has been washed with ordinary clean water, washing it with a salt solution may help prevent infection.

Liquid antiseptics

The advantage of liquid antiseptics is that they can be used to help wash a wound clean but they do not leave a greasy smear behind to interfere with normal healing processes. The two biggest-selling liquid antiseptics are probably *TCP Liquid Antiseptic* and *Dettol,* although there is also a *Savlon Antiseptic Liquid.*

Betadine consists of a type of iodine. *Dettol* contains chloroxylenol. *Hibitane* consists of chlorhexidine gluconate. *Savlon Antiseptic Liquid* contains chlorhexidine gluconate and cetrimide and *TCP Liquid Antiseptic* contains chlorine, phenol, iodine and salicylic acid. (There is also a *TCP First Aid Gel* which contains the liquid antiseptic in a gel basis.) *Betadine* is also available as an aerosol spray, a gargle and mouthwash, an ointment, a scalp and skin cleanser, a shampoo, a skin cleanser foam, a vaginal douche, a vaginal gel, vaginal pessaries and an antiseptic paint, and these different preparations are all based on the same formula.

There isn't much to choose between any of these antiseptic liquids. They are all useful for cleaning wounds, grazes, cuts and abrasions and although they won't by any means eradicate all infecting organisms they will almost certainly do more good than harm. I suggest you choose the cheapest.

Incidentally, anyone who watches cowboy films will know that alcohol can also be used as a liquid antiseptic. Personally, I would prefer to allow my alcohol to work from the inside but I suppose that in an emergency it could be used to help clean a dirty wound. If you get a cut while trapped in a Spanish airport, for example, you may be wiser to wash the wound with duty-free alcohol than with water.

Iodine solutions are excellent antiseptics but they usually stain everything brown and so are not popular with white-skinned people.

Antiseptic creams
There are hundreds and hundreds of different antiseptics used in the many creams that are available for use at home. To list them, differentiate between them, and to review their individual properties and disadvantages would take up several hundred pages and prove very boring. It would also be a complete waste of time since I do not intend to recommend any of them.

Cetrimide is one of the most popular antiseptics for use in antiseptic creams. It is inactivated by soap and may cause skin problems if used repeatedly. It is the basis of *Bactrian Antiseptic Cream, Cetavlon, Cetrimax Antiseptic Cream, Family Antiseptic Cream, Medicaid, Savlon Antiseptic Cream* and *Sterling Health Antiseptic Cream.*

Acriflex contains 0.1% aminacrine hydrochloride which is a disinfectant. This product is useful for the treatment of infected wounds or burns, but according to *Martindale's Extra Pharmacopoeia* it can delay healing if used for prolonged periods.

PHisoHex contains 0.75% hexachlorophane which is a useful disinfectant but which should not be used on damaged skin or on large areas of skin. According to *Martindale's*: 'central nervous stimulation and convulsions have occurred after absorption of hexachlorophane from burns and damaged skin'.

Many well-known, highly popular antiseptic creams contain a number of different substances. There is, in fact, an increased chance of developing an allergic reaction to a cream which has a number of constituents if the cream is used for a prolonged period.

Germolene Antiseptic Ointment, one of the biggest-selling products, contains ten substances when served up in a tin, and nine when sold in a tube. Other compound antiseptic creams include *Ayrton's Antiseptic Cream, Boots Antiseptic Cream, Boots Family Antiseptic, Exa-mol Antiseptic Ointment, Germ Ointment, Maws Junior Antiseptic Cream,* TCP *Ointment* and *Wright's Coal Tar Ointment.*

Incidentally, the advertisements for *Germolene* suggest that the cream is not only useful for cuts, scratches, grazes and spots, but also for blisters and chapped and rough skin. I don't think there is any point in putting an antiseptic cream or ointment on to skin which is rough rather than infected.

Antiseptic creams are also advertised as being useful for stings. *DDD Cream,* for example, which is advertised as containing five antiseptics, is said to be the thing for stings and bites. There is no need to use cream with one, two, three, four or five antiseptics in it when you've been bitten or stung, unless infection has occurred as a result of scratching.

Cleansing tissues

If you get cut or grazed far away from running water cleansing tissues might well be a good idea. These consist of saturated swabs which are packed in small sealed envelopes. Medicated versions include *Antiseptic Wipes* which are impregnated with cetrimide and isopropanolol, *Bidex Cleansing Tissues* which contain chlorhexidine gluconate and cetrimide and *Medi-swabs* (which consist of cotton-felt saturated with 70% isopropyl alcohol).

Sprays

These days almost everything is obtainable in an aerosol or spray can. For example, *Bidex Spray* contains chlorhexidine hydrochloride. Since much of the value in using an antiseptic cream lies in the rubbing and cleaning rather than the cream itself, it does seem to me that antiseptic sprays are rather pointless. They are also an expensive way to apply antiseptics to skin, furniture and friends. Incidentally, sprays intended for use by people with muscular aches have exactly the same disadvantage – it is the rubbing that often helps.

Ointments to promote healing

There are several ointments to help promote natural healing processes. *Antipeol* and *St James Balm* contain very similar ingredients: zinc oxide, ichthammol, salicylic acid and urea. *Boots Pink Healing Ointment* contains zinc oxide, methyl salicylate, liquefied phenol and menthol.

I can see no reason why any of these ointments should assist in the repair of damaged skin.

Plasters and dressings

Sticking plasters can be useful. If you have a cut and you want to do something messy or dirty, a plaster can provide protection. If you have a graze or sore spot that you keep knocking a plaster can help guard against further damage. Plasters can help hold together the two edges of a small cut while initial healing takes place.

But sticking plasters can also delay healing. Waterproof plasters which seal off a wound prevent natural recovery and medicated plasters do nothing to speed up healing.

Choosing a sticking plaster shouldn't be too difficult. The only really important criterion is price. Individually wrapped plasters are better because they're less likely to become infected before they are used. A box of assorted sizes gives you some choice. Medicated plasters (such as *Germolene Medicated Plasters*) are not worth buying, since in my view, the only useful purpose for a sticking plaster is to provide mechanical protection.

Use a plaster for short-term protection but take it off as soon as you can.

Bruises

If a blood vessel is damaged but the skin isn't broken and the blood which escapes from the broken blood vessel can't get out of your body the result is a bruise. The official medical term for a bruise, by the way, is an ecchymosis. It is the accumulating blood which causes both the swelling and discolouration associated with a bruise.

There are products on the market which are sold to help treat bruises. Most, such as *Bruzoff*, contain an antiseptic. Other treatments include the use of leeches, which suck out the accumulating blood and reduce the swelling, and such old-fashioned remedies as the application of raw steak.

A cold compress applied to the injury site before the bruise develops may produce vasoconstriction and therefore reduce the amount of swelling. Otherwise there is not much to be done.

Burns

Nine out of ten of the really serious burns which involve people in their own homes are caused by clothes catching fire. Once a dress or nightdress is burning there is a very great risk of the person wearing that piece of clothing being severely burned. So try to prevent burns.

Make sure that children's clothing, particularly night clothing which tends to be loose and therefore easy to drag against a fire, is made of non-inflammable material. Little girls may look prettier in nightdresses but they are safer in pyjamas if you have an open fire in the house.

Keep hot liquids, kettles and teapots well out of reach of small children. Despite many warnings thousands of children are burned each year by reaching up on to a table and pulling a vessel containing hot fluid over themselves. These burns can often be very damaging.

When someone is burnt put out any flames by wrapping the patient up tightly in a coat or blanket. Then cool them down as quickly as you can. The obvious way to do this is by immersing them in water. Run a bath or shower and keep the burned parts covered with cold water for ten minutes. Do this before calling for help. If you can cool down the burned parts you may help reduce the amount of damage. If there isn't a bath or shower handy use a cold compress or ice pack.

There are a number of myths about ways to cope with burns. Let me deal with some of the best-known.

Do not put butter or any other sort of oil on a burn. It won't help and may make things worse.

Do not cover a burn with a cottonwool dressing. Little bits of cotton-wool will stick to the burn and have to be picked off piece by piece. It isn't necessary to cover a burn as a first-aid measure.

Do not open any blisters which form. Leave them alone and try not to burst them.

It is worthwhile being able to differentiate between a first degree burn and a second degree burn.

A first degree burn may be extremely painful but it won't cause scarring and it will usually heal by itself. The skin is reddened but not blistered. Sunburns and scalds caused by steam are usually first degree burns.

First-aid treatment of a superficial, first degree burn is extremely simple. All you need to do is to keep cold running water on the burned tissues for five or ten minutes and then leave the burn alone.

A second degree burn always blisters. The blisters are caused by the accumulation of fluid from the blood vessels deep in the tissue which have been damaged by the burn. If treated carefully second degree burns can still heal by themselves and shouldn't produce scars. A fairly small second degree burn can be treated at home. Clean the skin by patting with a gauze pad that has been dipped into a liquid antiseptic. Then cover it with a clean, dry dressing. Wrap the dressing on fairly firmly. If clothing is stuck to the burn then you must see a doctor. It is, incidentally, a good idea to remove all rings and bracelets if it is a hand that is burnt. Fingers may swell up later. Examine the burned area daily and if you are not certain that it is healing well then ask for advice.

If you haven't any sterile dressings then use recently washed and ironed handkerchiefs or teatowels. Make sure that the material doesn't moult. If it does the little bits of cloth will stick to the burn.

Any type of burn that is more serious than the ones I have described is a third degree burn and you will definitely need professional help. If the skin is obviously severely damaged then it is essential to get the patient to hospital as soon as possible. A second degree burn that has affected more than two or three square inches of skin should be seen by a doctor.

There are many branded creams available for the treatment of burns. Most contain an antiseptic. *Aidex Burn and Wound Cream*, *Ayrtons Burn Cream* and *Cupal Burn Aid* all contain aminacrine (see p.98).

Burneze is an aerosol which contains mepyramine maleate and benzocaine. Mepyramine maleate is an antihistamine and benzocaine is a local anaesthetic.

I suggest that you stick to the simpler methods of treatment I have described.

When to ask for medical advice
If a cut or wound bleeds profusely or doesn't stop bleeding within half an hour it should be attended to by a doctor. Any cut which is more than an inch long will certainly need stitching as will any cut which gapes and which cannot be held together with sticking plaster. Smaller cuts on the hands or face should be attended to by a professional since careful stitching can reduce the amount of subsequent scarring.

A superficial burn which involves more than two or three square inches of skin should be seen by a doctor. Any burn which has caused such severe damage that there is bleeding or weeping from it should be attended to professionally.

CYSTITIS
The symptoms of cystitis vary. Sometimes a sufferer complains that she is always rushing off to the toilet to pass urine and finding, when she's got there, that it's been a false alarm. And sometimes the complaint is about a stinging when the urine is passed. I've said 'she' because although men do get cystitis it is far more common among women. There is no subtle hormonal explanation for this variation. The explanation is simple and anatomical: in women the urethra (the tube which connects the bladder to the outside world) is shorter, more vulnerable and less of a problem for invading infective organisms.

Infections are one of the common causes of cystitis and there are several things that can be done to minimize this risk. The experts say that frequent bathing is useful and that plain, simple soaps should be used in preference to disinfectants or strongly perfumed soaps which can, in fact, make things worse. Cotton, rather than nylon, underwear and loose-fitting clothes help prevent the breeding of infective organisms. Stockings are said to be better than tights for the woman who is prone to cystitis.

Sex is another common cause of cystitis since the female urethra may be bruised or damaged by some positions. To prevent this type of problem (known rather quaintly as 'honeymoon cystitis') all you can do is avoid uncomfortable or painful positions and use a plain lubricant to reduce soreness and pain. *K-Y Lubricating Jelly* seems to be the most widely acceptable product for this problem.

If despite these simple precautions you still get an attack of cystitis there is much that you can do to minimize the symptoms.

To help flush out any infection you need to drink as much water as you can manage. You really do need to drink several glasses of water every hour. It may sound a crazy treatment for someone whose complaint is that they are finding passing urine painful but the explanation is simply that by drinking you'll be helping to wash out the infection.

You can relieve some of the stinging or burning and at the same time help kill off some of any bugs which may be involved by putting a teaspoonful of sodium bicarbonate (baking soda) into a glass of water or squash and drinking it. The sodium bicarbonate makes the urine slightly less acid and bacteria don't like this. There are plenty of other products which you can use to do this but most of them are more expensive and baking soda should be present in your home medicine chest (see p.193) for its value as an emergency antacid.

Repeat the dose of baking soda once an hour for three hours. You can use any painkiller you like (see p.134) and most people find that the warmth of a hot-water bottle (see p.141) placed over the bladder is most helpful.

If the symptoms persist for more than five days or don't seem to be improving after twenty-four hours then see your own doctor. Incidentally don't be too worried if your urine contains blood and looks red or smoky coloured – this is a common symptom and usually means nothing of significance. For the sake of safety, however, see your doctor if you see or think you see blood in your urine.

DANDRUFF

Dandruff isn't so much a problem involving the hair as a disorder of the scalp, and like so many other skin problems it's a trouble that frequently recurs. It often starts at the age of ten and continues to cause showers of trouble for decades afterwards, the small white scales often being accompanied by an itching of the scalp which simply heightens the associated embarrassment.

Dermatologists recognize two types of dandruff. In the first type the dandruff occurs on an oily, greasy scalp. In the second it affects the individual with dry, brittle hair. In both types the dandruff scales originate from the superficial layer of the skin where there is some disorder in the rate at which dead cells flake away from the protective layer of cells on the skin's surface.

Dandruff may seem to be more of a social and cosmetic problem than a medical one but it is still a disorder which needs treatment. The important point to remember is that treatment usually needs to be regular rather than erratic and initiated when dandruff recurs.

There are several useful drugs available for the treatment of dandruff.

Selenium sulphide is an effective shampoo ingredient. It is a powerful chemical which is extremely dangerous if taken by mouth. It is so toxic that it should not be used on inflamed areas of skin, it should not be allowed to enter the eyes, and it should not be used indefinitely. If it is used for long periods of time (three months or more) it can cause a temporary hair loss.

When using a product containing selenium sulphide the scalp is first washed with soap and water and then rinsed. After rinsing with clean water 5–10 ml of shampoo containing 2.5% selenium sulphide is applied together with a small amount of warm water. The resultant lather is rinsed off and the application of shampoo repeated. This time the lather should be left on the hair for five minutes at least. This is the point where most people lose patience and abandon their treatment too quickly. After treatment the hair should be well rinsed and the hands and nails cleaned well.

The shampooing needs to be done twice a week for two weeks and then once a week for another two weeks. After that the shampoo can be used when it is needed.

Selenium sulphide is available as *Lenium, Selenium Sulphide Scalp Application BPC* and *Selsun.*

Another equally useful dandruff shampoo constituent is zinc pyrithione. Products which contain 1% zinc pyrithione include *Head and Shoulders* and *Revlon ZP11 Formula Medicated Shampoo.*

There are, of course, other shampoos available and the constituents of these vary a great deal. Many contain antiseptics and disinfectants. For example, *Banish Shampoo, Betadine Shampoo, Dandricide, Prodan Dandruff Treatment, Torbetol Shampoo* and *Vaseline Medicated Shampoo* all contain certain ingredients in this general category.

Salicylic acid and precipitated sulphur are both constituents of *Dr Page Barker's Dandruff Lotion* and methyl salicylate is an ingredient of *Gill's Dandruff Remover.* Both these can help remove the superficial layer of dead skin cells, while coal tar, which is an ingredient of *Sebbix Liquid Shampoo, Tegrin Shampoo* and *Vosene,* can also help to improve the condition of the scalp.

There are also a number of more imaginative preparations for the treatment or prevention of dandruff. These include *Epigran,* a wheat germ scalp tonic, *Juniper and Buckwheat Shampoo* and *Nettle Extract Anti-Dandruff Lotion.*

The choice of an ordinary shampoo must largely be dictated by personal preference and cosmetic requirements, but if dandruff is the problem then a shampoo containing either selenium sulphide or zinc pyrithione is probably the best buy. If one of these substances does not work then I suggest that a doctor's advice is sought. There are more powerful products which can be prescribed.

DIARRHOEA

Diarrhoea, in common with constipation, is difficult to define accurately. Because there is no such thing as a normal bowel habit what may seem to be an attack of diarrhoea to one individual may, when experienced by another, be described as a bout of constipation.

Diarrhoea is usually defined in medical textbooks as 'frequent, loose stools'. But that three-word definition includes two subjective assessments. I think it is probably wisest to assume that any increase in the frequency of bowel movements can be described as diarrhoea. Together with that assumption we must make another: that only attacks of 'diarrhoea' which prove inconvenient rather than simply exceptional should be treated.

The commonest two causes of diarrhoea are stress and gastro-intestinal infections.

Stress, anxiety, worry, nervousness – call it what you like – is a common reason for a brief, short-lived bout of diarrhoea. Soldiers suffer before a battle, students before examinations, sportsmen before events, brides before weddings, job applicants before interviews. This type of diarrhoea isn't usually worth treating for the very good reason that it will frequently have cleared up in a matter of hours. If it does persist for more than a few hours and it is definitely caused by stress a bottle of anti-diarrhoeal mixture is unlikely to be the best solution to the problem. Learning to relax is more likely to provide a lasting solution (see my book *Stress Control*).

When a bout of diarrhoea is caused by an infection there are likely to be clues to the cause. If other members of the family have the same disorder then the cause is likely to be something that has been eaten. If the sufferer has just returned from a trip away from home (not necessarily abroad) then the diarrhoea may have been caused by an infection contracted as a result of lower-than-usual standards of hygiene. If the diarrhoea was preceded by vomiting then once again food poisoning is a likely explanation.

There is a third common cause of diarrhoea which is well worth mentioning. It is, I'm afraid, often a fact that doctors cause diarrhoea with the pills they prescribe for infections in other parts of the body. These pills (such as penicillin) kill off the bugs which normally live in the bowel and allow other bugs to make their presence felt. When the prescribed drug is stopped the diarrhoea will usually clear up by itself. If you are taking a prescribed drug and you suspect that it may be causing your diarrhoea don't just stop taking it – telephone the doctor who prescribed the drug and ask for advice. It may be better for you to persevere and treat the diarrhoea as well than to abandon your course and allow the original infection to recur. In addition to antibiotics other drugs can cause diarrhoea – antacids and health salts are common culprits.

Finally, there are three other common types of diarrhoea. Firstly, there is the partygoer who eats too much or drinks too much and whose diarrhoea is a fairly understandable consequence of this over-indulgence. Secondly, there is the child who has a chest infection or an ear infection and who develops diarrhoea as a symptomatic bonus. The diarrhoea will usually disappear as the main infection clears up. And thirdly, there is the patient who regularly takes a laxative and who has persistent diarrhoea as a direct result of this bad habit. This may sound bizarre but it is by no means an infrequent occurrence.

Whatever the cause of your diarrhoea the treatment is likely to be very much the same. For twenty-four hours avoid food but remember that it is important to ensure that you do not become dehydrated. Frequent bursts of diarrhoea can result in considerable fluid losses and it is vital to make sure that the lost fluid is replaced. This may be the only action necessary. Symptomatic relief can be obtained by the use of any one of the substances recommended below.

The medicines available for the treatment of diarrhoea fall into several categories.

To begin with there are the drugs which form a bulky mass inside the bowel and help carry away irritants as they are excreted. Kaolin, aluminium hydroxide and other aluminium salts, pectin, bismuth salts, calcium carbonate and activated charcoal fall into this category.

Then there are the drugs which act on the bowel wall – slowing down the movements which result in diarrhoea. Because they act on the muscle walls these drugs may also relieve the griping pains associated with diarrhoea. Drugs in this group include the opiates, such as morphine and the anticholinergic drugs. (Before the mention of morphine conjures up visions of setting up a local drug ring I should point out there isn't very much morphine in a bottle of anti-diarrhoeal mixture and it is mixed up with kaolin. Morphine and kaolin mixture can therefore be described as both legal and binding.)

Thirdly, there are drugs like iodochlorhydroxyquin (otherwise known as clioquinol) which are intended to help eradicate invading bacteria and thereby prevent or treat infective diarrhoea.

Some products contain a mixture of substances from each of these categories. These combination therapies are unlikely to contain enough of anything to be helpful.

Finally, remember that when you start eating again after a bout of diarrhoea it is wise to begin with foods which provide roughage – dry toast and bran may help, for example. The right food may be more helpful than any medicine.

Kaolin and morphine

Kaolin is the commonest constituent of anti-diarrhoeal mixtures. Its chemical name is aluminium silicate and its value is that when given by mouth it absorbs toxic substances from the intestinal tract, increases the bulk of the faeces and helps the body get rid of irritant substances with less discomfort and less delay than might otherwise be the case.

The best way to buy kaolin is as *Kaolin Mixture BPC*. About 20 ml of this should be taken four or five times a day to slow down a diarrhoeal attack. The kaolin needs to be freshly prepared. There is also a *Paediatric Kaolin Mixture BPC* which is perfectly suitable for children and which should be given in 5 or 10 ml doses according to age. Children over the age of five or six can be given a half-dose of ordinary *Kaolin Mixture BPC*.

Most of the anti-diarrhoeal mixtures available which contain kaolin also contain other substances. *Boots Diarrhoea Mixture* contains kaolin and aluminium hydroxide gel. *Woodward's Diarrhoea Mixture* contains kaolin and apple pectin. *Sterling Health Anti-Diarrhoeal Mixture* contains just ordinary kaolin.

Adults Diarrhoea Mixture contains an impressive-sounding mixture of kaolin, calcium carbonate, clioquinol, cinnamon oil, nutmeg oil, clove oil and cardamom oil. *Carmil* contains pectin, kaolin, morphine hydrochloride and atropine methonitrate. *Enterosan Tablets* contain camomile, kaolin, morphine hydrochloride, sorbitol, belladonna tincture and peppermint oil. *Savory and Moore Sickness and Diarrhoea Mixture* contains kaolin, pectin, peppermint oil, chloroform and belladonna. I do not recommend any of these products because I see no advantage in using multiple mixtures.

Diatabs and *Diocalm Tablets* both contain morphine hydrochloride and a kaolin-like substance. Since they are available in a more convenient form they are obviously of use to travellers who might find carrying a bottle of kaolin or kaolin and morphine inconvenient.

J. Collis Browne's mixture

This product has been on sale for over a century and is advertised for use by people with coughs as well as those with diarrhoea. The reason for this 'double value' is simple – the compound contains morphine which has an effect on both symptoms. In addition to morphine the constituents are chloroform, spirit, capsicum extract, peppermint oil and glycerol.

This mixture has been diluted in recent years and its present morphine content is so low that anyone hoping to satisfy a craving for morphine would need to buy and drink several bottles a day.

As an anti-diarrhoeal medicine I cannot see any particular reason to recommend this mixture.

Clioquinol

A few years ago just about everyone going abroad used to carry a box of magic anti-diarrhoeal tablets. And, of course, anyone taking these tablets who didn't get diarrhoea would swear by the effectiveness of the product.

The usual basic constituent of those tablets (the most widely known of which was probably *Entero-Vioform*) was clioquinol. In a previous book of mine, *The Medicine Men*, I described how the dangers associated with this product have become apparent and why it ought not to be offered for general sale. The disease with which clioquinol has been associated, Asian subacute myelo-optic neuropathy, was first recognized in the late 1950s and since then over 10,000 people have been diagnosed as having it in Japan alone. It is perhaps enough to say that the Committee on Safety of Medicines has recently advised that this product should be available only on prescription, and in my experience it is not often prescribed.

At the time of writing this book clioquinol is still available in some home medicines. Before buying any brand name anti-diarrhoeal read the label carefully. Don't buy anything which contains this substance.

Holiday diarrhoea

Every year thousands of holidaymakers have their expensive days in the sun ruined by what they may later wryly refer to as 'Spanish tummy'. Most of these physically wearing and socially disastrous incidents could have been avoided not by consuming large quantities of protective medicines (which do not help and may be dangerous) but by following some simple basic rules while abroad.

The first mistake which many people make is to leap off the aeroplane and immediately start downing vast quantities of local food and washing it down with litres of rough, local wine. After such outrageous insults diarrhoea is not only inevitable, it is also deserved. It may be the only way that the human body can hope to cope with what may be an unprecedented problem. If you're going abroad, or even travelling in your own country, then eat and drink in moderation for the first two or three days to give your body a chance to adapt.

If you are staying in an area renowned for stomach upsets and you suspect that the drinking water is not thoroughly purified, then drink only bottled water. Having decided to do that remember to clean your teeth with bottled water, to throw ice cubes out of drinks, to avoid freshly washed salads and fruit that you cannot peel yourself and to avoid ice-creams that are not packed in individual wrappers bearing the name of a reputable manufacturer.

Should these precautions prove unsuccessful and you do develop diarrhoea starve for twenty-four hours and drink plenty of bottled fluids. See the list on p.193 for details of medicines to take with you when travelling abroad.

Conclusion

Do drink plenty of fluids if you get diarrhoea – fruit squash is fine and has the advantage that you can add a pinch of salt without making yourself sick. This helps because salt depletion following diarrhoea can result in faintness. Other useful replacement fluids include *Bovril*, *Marmite* and *Oxo*, all of which contain essential sodium. There is even good sense in drinking a cup of clear chicken broth – an old family remedy.

Do not eat until the diarrhoea has begun to settle. Then start off by eating bland foods which give plenty of bulk. If you eat very hot, spicy food while you're recovering you must expect the diarrhoea to return.

If the diarrhoea is particularly unpleasant or troublesome and you want to get out and about a little while you're suffering and recovering try *Kaolin Mixture BPC* or *Kaolin and Morphine Mixture BPC*. Don't expect to feel fit and lively for a day or two even if the diarrhoea has slowed down.

See a doctor if the diarrhoea continues for more than five days, if it's accompanied by severe abdominal pain, is accompanied by bleeding or keeps on recurring. Diarrhoea can be a symptom of a threatening disease. And any potentially dangerous disease is easier to deal with when diagnosed early.

Note If you regularly take a prescribed medicine and you have an attack of diarrhoea the pills you're taking may not have a chance to be properly absorbed. Ask your doctor if you're worried. A woman taking the contraceptive pill should consider herself unprotected for the rest of her cycle if she has diarrhoea after or while taking her pill.

EAR DISORDERS

As a general rule I do not recommend home treatment for ear disorders. It is certainly not wise to put drops of any kind into a painful ear or to attempt to remove wax with any probe or scraping device. The ear drum is too easily damaged.

In an emergency, of course, aspirin and paracetamol tablets (see p.134) can be used for treating earache but any persistent earache needs to be investigated by a doctor.

Deafness is another problem which should not be dealt with unless professional advice has been sought. There are a number of companies selling hearing aids today but in Britain anyone who suffers from deafness is entitled to free treatment. Modern hearing aids provided through the health service are not necessarily as cumbersome, unsightly and ineffective as many people believe. Anyone suffering from hearing loss should seek medical advice and only consider purchasing an aid if health service aids seem unsuitable.

The other common problem associated with the ears is wax. This is a frequent cause of deafness and dizziness. There are a number of proprietary preparations (*Cerumol, Earex, Waxsol,* etc.) designed to soften and help in the removal of wax. Unfortunately, even after the use of drops syringing may be needed if all the wax is to be effectively removed. If you're sure that your problem is caused by wax try using one of the preparations mentioned (or ordinary olive oil) and then visit your doctor after five days if there has been no improvement. Any wax that may be there will then be fairly easy to remove by syringing.

EYE DISORDERS

Never buy anything to put into your eyes. If you have any eye symptoms which persist then see a doctor.

Having damned a multimillion-pound market in twenty words let me explain why.

There are many reasons why your eyes may be red, sticky, sore, itchy or painful. Ninety-nine times out of a hundred it is possible to treat a minor eye problem quickly and easily with a bottle of drops or a tube of eye ointment but on the hundredth occasion such simple treatment will not solve the problem. And if expert advice from an opthalmic surgeon is not sought on that one occasion the sight may be damaged permanently. It's a risk that just is not worth taking.

Of course, there will be many times when eye symptoms will clear up quickly and without any treatment being needed. If you have been sitting in a dry, dusty atmosphere – perhaps thick with cigarette smoke – and your eyes become red and sore as a result, they will quickly return to normal when you get out of the dust and smoke. If you have sore, itchy, red eyes which get worse when you're out in the open in the pollen season then you may simply be exhibiting signs of hay fever. Some people don't sneeze or get any nasal symptoms at all. These eye symptoms can be relieved by avoiding the open air when the pollen count is at its highest and by wearing sunglasses (see p.161). If neither of these precautions are practicable, however, then see a doctor.

Eye infections are extremely common. The usual symptoms of conjunctivitis (an infection of the conjunctiva – the thin membrane which lines the eyelids and covers the eyeball) are a grittiness in the eye which usually feels as though there is something in it, and a stickiness which is worse on waking. It may sometimes seem as though the eyelids are glued together. If gently bathing the eyes in clean warm water doesn't clear the infection away then a doctor can prescribe the appropriate treatment. Conjunctivitis is extremely infectious and it is important not to use the same face cloth or towel on an uninfected eye. If you do the infection will spread. It can quite quickly affect all the members of a household if a communal towel is used.

Styes are small, infected spots which occur around the eyes. Any pus which comes out should be wiped away carefully and the whole area bathed with clean warm water. If you use an eye bath do make sure that it is sterilized properly after use. Put it in boiling water. If it isn't heat

resistant and it cracks then you're probably better off without it anyway. A stye which doesn't get better and go away needs to be seen by a
doctor. Don't try treating it at home.

There is one other common eye problem that can be cured without
any treatment. It's one that mostly affects women since it's relatively
unusual for men to use eye makeup. If the eye becomes red and itchy
and you use a lot of eye makeup or have recently changed to a different
brand, then try leaving off eye makeup altogether for a few days. If
the problem clears up you've found the cause. The solution is obvious.
There are, incidentally, cosmetic products available which are specially
formulated for women who tend to develop allergic rashes to ordinary
products.

Eye drops, lotions and ointments

Phenylephrine hydrochloride (the product so popular among the
manufacturers of cold remedies) is a common constituent of eye
remedies. It constricts the dilated blood vessels in a red eye and so
reduces the amount of redness; it also helps to dilate the pupil. The
following products contain this drug: *Degest, Eyeclear Eye Drops,
Eyesoothe Eye Lotion, Optabs* and *Steri-fresh*. These products may be safe
for very short-term use but they become dangerous when reapplied
again and again as the effect wears off and the redness recurs. *Optabs*
also contain adrenalin to reduce conjunctival congestion. *Murine Eye
Drops* contain naphazoline hydrochloride which has a similar effect and
Collyre Bleu Laiter contains naphazoline nitrate.

By far the biggest-selling eye care preparations in Britain are *Optrex
Eye Lotion* and *Optrex Eye Ointment* which contain a number of antiseptics. *Optrex Eye Lotion* contains witch hazel, boric acid, salicylic
acid, chlorbutol and zinc sulphate. *Optrex Eye Ointment* contains
gramicidin and aminacrine hydrochloride. A third Optrex product
called *Optone Eye Drops* contains witch hazel, borax and chlorbutol.

Other products which contain mixtures of astringents, disinfectants
and antiseptics include *Boots Eye Drops, Lanes Eye Lotion, Pennine Eye
Drops* and *Visimax Eye Lotion*.

I do not recommend any of these products for the reasons I have
already explained at the beginning of this section.

All eye products should, if used at all, be used strictly according to the instructions since overuse can be hazardous. Most manufacturers warn customers not to use eye drops, ointments or lotions if symptoms persist. In the absence of more specific instructions I suggest that no eye symptoms should be treated for more than five days without expert advice being sought.

Lyteers is a well-known artificial tear solution for those who find real tears unobtainable and fresh water uncomfortable. Finally, there are the *Simhealth Eyes Right Capsules* which contain vitamin A (see p.180).

Artificial eyes
Patients with artificial eyes should normally consult their own doctor or an ophthalmic specialist if they have any problems. Special lubricants (such as *Solpro*) are available for use with artificial eyes.

Sunglasses (see p.161)

Contact lenses
These days more and more people are wearing contact lenses instead of spectacles. Lenses can be divided into two main categories – soft or hard – according to the materials from which they are manufactured. There are a number of products available for use with contact lenses while they are in the eye and when they need cleaning.

I would strongly suggest that readers should accept the advice of their opticians when choosing products for use with contact lenses. For the sake of completeness I have compiled a list of some of the products which are available.

Products for the care, cleansing and storing of soft contact lenses include *Barnes-Hind Cleaner No. 4, Hexidin, Hydrocare Protein Remover, Hydrosoak, Hydrosol, Monoclens, Pliacide, Pliagel, Salette, Steri-lette, Steri-Sal, Steri-soft* and *Steri-solv*.

For cleaning, wetting, soaking and storing hard contact lenses the following products are available: *Barnes-Hind Cleaning and Soaking Solution, Barnes-Hind Comfort Drops, Barnes-Hind Gel Clean, Barnes-Hind One Solution, Barnes-Hind Wetting Solution, Blink N Clean, Clean-N-Soak, Contacare, Contactasoak, Contactasol, LC 65, Lens-Mate, Soakare, Soquette, Steri-clens, Steri-soak, Titan, Total* and *Transol*.

When to see a doctor
You should see a doctor as soon as possible if you lose your eyesight temporarily or permanently, partially or totally. You should also see a doctor as a matter of some urgency if you have a severe pain in or around the eye.

FOOT PROBLEMS
It is estimated that nine out of ten people have foot problems of one sort or another. When you realize how badly most people treat their feet, it is perhaps more surprising that there is one faultless pair in ten than that there are nine pairs giving trouble.

There is much that can be done to minimize foot trouble. Wearing comfortable shoes that fit properly and provide the necessary support is a help. Cutting toenails regularly and carefully also helps, and washing and drying the feet daily can help prevent skin troubles on the feet.

There are a number of problems which involve the feet. Warts and verrucae are discussed on p.188, and chilblains on p.70; corns, callouses and hard skin, infections such as 'athlete's foot' and ingrowing toenails are discussed in this section.

Corns and callouses
Corns and callouses are caused by a thickening of the horny layer of the skin. A callous is a flat area of thickened skin, while a corn is an inverted, cone-shaped thickening. These can occur on the hands, feet or any other part of the body which is regularly rubbed. On the feet, corns are often caused by badly fitting shoes, shoes which are made of hard, unbending materials, shoes with pointed toes or with very high heels.

Corns and callouses can be treated at home quite effectively. The affected skin should first be soaked in warm water for a few minutes and then rubbed with a rough towel, soapstone or emery board to remove loosened tissue. It is never wise to cut or pick at the skin however hard it may seem. Infected areas may take months to heal.

There are a number of special devices available for rubbing at hardened skin. *Miracle Stone, Newton's Chiropody Sponge* and *Scholl Hard*

Skin Reducer can be used for this purpose. I don't recommend knives, planes or any cutting instruments for use at home.

As either an adjunct or alternative to these devices one of the proprietary corn creams or ointments can be applied to continue the treatment. *Ayrtons Corn and Wart Paint, Boots Corn Paint, Carnation Corn Paint, Diamond Corn Solvent, Dispello Corn Cure, Freezone, Hiker Corn Salve, Pickles Ointment for Hard Skin, Scholl Corn and Callous Salve, Three Flasks Corn and Wart Solvent* and *Union Jack Corn Plasters* all contain salicylic acid which is a keratolytic. It is important not to allow these creams or ointments to be rubbed on to healthy skin since they may cause damage. They are, after all, intended to help soften and remove offending hard skin. Special 'corn plasters' which are impregnated with salicylic acid include *Amovon Corn Caps, Carnation Corn Caps, Scholl Zino Corn Pads* and *Union Jack Corn Plasters*. These help to ensure that the salicylic acid is retained on or near to the corn or callous and also help to cushion sore points. *Salicylic Acid Collodion BPC* and *Salicylic Acid Paint* can also be obtained. *Scholl Air Pillo Insoles, Scholls Cosy Sole Insoles* and *Omniped Foot Cushions* can help prevent the development of hard skin.

Athlete's foot (see also **Ringworm** p.190)
Athlete's foot is a highly contagious fungal infection which thrives in warm, wet conditions. Symptoms which include an itchy rash, blisters on the skin and splits between the toes are made worse when the feet sweat in hot weather. There are several useful products available. *Balto Athlete's Foot Lotion, Mycil Ointment, Mycil Powder, Scholl Athlete's Foot Powder* and *Scholl S1 Athlete's Foot Liquid* should all be effective. Treatment should be continued for several days after the symptoms have subsided, and to prevent a recurrence it is wise not to walk barefoot in public showers, baths or swimming pools. Advice that is easier to give than to take!

Ingrowing toenails
Ingrowing toenails can cause a tremendous amount of pain. The best way to avoid the problem is to ensure that toenails are cut regularly, but not too short. It is also important to cut the nails straight across so

that the corners of the newly-growing nail do not grow into the flesh. Treating the problem usually requires expert advice either from a chiropodist or a doctor, although Scholl do make an *Ingrown Toenail Treatment* which might be worth trying as long as there is no sign of infection at the site.

Scholl, incidentally, also make an enormous range of cushions, supports, liners, grips, props, separators, pads, shields and plasters designed to relieve pressure on painful parts of the feet. These can provide symptomatic relief and, by temporarily relieving pressure, speed healing.

There are a great many other foot products. Scholl make an *Antiseptic Foot Balm, Dry Powder Antiperspirant Spray, Foot Deodorant Spray* and *Foot Refresher Spray*. There is also *Germolene Medicated Foot Spray, Healthy Feet Cream, Healthy Feet Spray* and *Valpeda Foot Balm*. Some of these products are designed to keep feet feeling fresh, and others to stop unpleasant odours developing.

Most of these products need to be used as cosmetics rather than for medicinal purposes. Avoiding nylon socks, wearing leather shoes, washing frequently and using an ordinary, plain talcum powder will probably be more effective in keeping down sweating than using deodorant or antiseptic creams or sprays.

If any foot condition persists, then advice should be sought either from a doctor or a chiropodist. Diabetics should never treat foot problems themselves and any ulceration which develops on the feet should be treated professionally.

HAIR LOSS

Despite an almost total lack of evidence in their favour and a surfeit of opinion opposing their continued production and promotion hair restoratives are probably as popular today as they have ever been. Indeed, baldness is one of the growing number of problems which today attracts the attention of companies specializing in the production of cosmetics as well as those which market medicines.

Before considering the value of hair restoratives it is necessary to examine the physiology of hair growth.

The basic and most important fact is that every single hair on your head has its own root; a root which was there when you were born and which produces a new hair from time to time. Not all the roots produce hairs at the same time and occasionally some roots may temporarily stop producing hairs.

As the years go by and more roots rest and stop producing hairs baldness develops. The chances of roots stopping hair production permanently at a relatively early age depend almost entirely upon an individual's genetic makeup. The genes which determine whether or not you'll go bald at thirty are as uncontrollable as the genes which determine your height and eye colour.

Genetically determined baldness affects men far more often than women and begins with a thinning of the hair above the temples and on top of the head. It gradually spreads over the scalp leaving a good growth around the sides and the back of the head. Men who don't like signs of developing baldness sometimes try to hide their shinier patches by combing long strands of hair from the sides over the centre.

The type of alopecia (a medical term for baldness) which causes most worry is that described by doctors as alopecia areata. In this condition the hair loss is both sudden and dramatic. Hair falls out in patches all over the scalp, coming out in handfuls as the roots suddenly stop growing in their thousands. It's a sort of hair root strike. This disorder most commonly affects young people in their teens and twenties and affects females as well as males. Doctors don't really know exactly what causes it but most suspect that it is exacerbated if not actually caused by worry or emotional strain. The most reassuring note about this disease is that within a few months most patients will have grown a full head of hair again. The magical hair restoratives which can provide anecdotal proof of patients having benefited might have been used on patients with this spontaneously resolving disorder.

There are, of course, other causes of baldness. Some powerful drugs, for example, can be responsible for hair loss as can infections of the scalp. But stories that baldness is related to the wearing or not of a hat, the type of shampoo used, or the climate have never been verified.

The remedies which are available over the chemist's counter or from home medicine manufacturers and wholesalers by mail contain a number of differing constituents. Since none of them seem to be based on scientific fact there is no logical way to assess their usefulness. Manufacturers sometimes advertise products as hair tonics, designed to produce healthier hair. These are as controversial as products advertised and sold as hair restoratives.

Several products contain vitamins – the universal panacea according to a number of promoters. *H Pantoten Hair Nutrition Tablets,* described as the 'unique vitamin formula for essential nutrition of hair and nails' contain vitamin H, iron, calcium pantothenate, vitamins F, B5 and B9, inositol and methionine. Inositol has been described as a curative for alopecia in mice but I can see no reason to recommend this product for humans. Nor can I see any reason why anyone eating a normal diet should benefit from taking *Head High Hair Vitamin Capsules* which contain 'specially selected vitamins and minerals vital to healthy hair'.

Gerovital H3 (Aslan) Hair Lotion is an expensive liquid said to be designed for the 'care and regeneration of the hair and for the prevention of hair loss' and contains as its active constituent a local anaesthetic called procaine hydrochloride. This is the basic ingredient of a substance sold as a rejuvenating agent. According to the 1978 edition of *Martindale's Extra Pharmacopoeia* the remarkable claims for this ingredient are not supported by any scientifically valid evidence or by the trials carried out independently.

Another product, *McKintol Hair Tonic,* contains benzoic acid, boric acid, thymol, chlorocresol and industrial methylated spirit. I'm not sure why a cocktail of disinfectants and antiseptics should be advertised as a hair tonic.

Old wives' tales for preventing and curing baldness
To prevent baldness developing try wearing an ivy leaf wreath. If the remedy fails, or is too late, try rubbing your scalp with a raw onion and then smearing the whole area with honey. If that is too messy for you try combing your hair the wrong way with a comb dipped in nettle juice, or sprinkle parsley seeds over your head three times a year.

These remedies are as likely to be effective as any proprietary medicines or expensive home cures!

HEADACHE (see also **Pain** p.134)
The commonest cause of a headache is tension. The man who has had a busy day at work, has been stuck in a traffic jam for two hours and

been worrying about a business deal will probably develop one. The woman who has been battling her way through crowded stores, who has missed her bus and been hurrying to get home before the children get in from school may have one. Tension headaches are a common sign that the stress threshold has been reached.

Tension headaches are caused by a sustained, painful contraction of the muscles around the face, scalp and neck. The headache, which usually seems throbbing and may affect any part of the head, will invariably disappear if the patient sits quietly for a while and perhaps takes a couple of mild analgesic tablets.

There are, of course, many other causes of headache. Headaches across the forehead, accompanied by a feeling of stuffiness and a difficulty in breathing are often caused by sinusitis and catarrh (see p.74). They may be worse in the morning, and are sometimes helped by a warm shower. These may need antibiotic tablets before they clear up. An infected or rotten tooth can cause a headache which seems to spread far beyond the area of tissue around the tooth (see p.176). Indeed, sometimes the pain seems to be completely unrelated to the tooth itself. The pain is transmitted by nerves which pass nearby the tooth. Toothache may merit a visit to the dentist, but if an infection is causing the problem you will probably have to take antibiotics before the tooth can be dealt with.

Very high blood pressure may cause headaches which are worse on waking and which are concentrated at the back of the head. People who, because of poor lighting conditions or poor eyesight, squint a great deal when reading or studying figures may develop headaches which are worse in the evenings and are concentrated at the front of the head. These headaches are caused by screwing up the muscles around the eyes. Ear infections cause headaches, usually around the ears.

Alcohol, of course, is also a cause of headaches. Mixing drinks is a sure way to develop a headache, although champagne alone is particularly liable to cause pains in the head. To avoid an alcohol-induced headache and the other accompanying feelings of being hungover drink plenty of water after a heavy consumption of alcohol.

Arthritis in the cervical spine, and the neck, is another common cause of headache. Less common causes include an inflammatory disease known as 'temporal arthritis' and the various types of brain tumour which are all rare. Meningitis, an uncommon inflammation of the covering over the brain, also causes headache and neck stiffness. Migraine, a common type of headache, is discussed elsewhere (see p.128). Finally, bumps and bangs on the head cause pain.

As I have said, the commonest cause of a headache is worry. Paradoxically the pains may well be at their worst when the problems which caused the worry have eased. Experts believe that this is because during relaxation the blood flow into the brain changes. In times of tension there is a decreased flow of blood into the brain caused probably by the tensing of muscles. When the muscles relax the blood flow increases. Most 'worry' headaches can be treated at home with soluble aspirin or paracetamol tablets (see p.134) and plenty of rest. But if a headache lasts more than a day, is accompanied by vomiting or follows a blow on the head then see a doctor.

INDIGESTION AND UPSET STOMACH

If five people sit down to dinner, one of them will suffer from indigestion afterwards. That, at least, is what the medical statisticians say and since a total of some £20 million a year is spent on antacid preparations it is difficult to argue with them.

Nearly half of all households have one of the dozens of available indigestion remedies in a cupboard somewhere. Since sales have risen by an average 27% each year since 1972, it seems likely that the number of indigestion remedies on the market is likely to continue rising. Selecting the right remedy will, therefore, become more and more difficult.

Milk of Magnesia and *Rennies* are currently among the market leaders, and sales of *Alka Seltzer, Andrews, BiSoDol, Macleans* and *Setlers* are also significant.

Before discussing the values of these and other medicines I'll explain what indigestion is, what causes it, what you can do to prevent it developing and when you must see a doctor about it.

The pains are usually confined to the centre of the chest and they often occur a short while after eating. They may be accompanied and even relieved by burping or bringing up wind. It's important to say right away that it is possible to confuse the pains of angina (early heart pain) with the pains of indigestion. Any chest pains which are brought on by exercise rather than eating, which are accompanied by breathlessness, or which also affect the arms and shoulders need to be treated by an expert.

There are several possible causes of indigestion. Sometimes the pains can be caused by simply eating or drinking too much or too quickly. Very spicy or fatty foods are particularly likely to cause indigestion.

Too much alcohol, tea or strong coffee can also cause indigestion as can smoking on an empty stomach. Worry is another causative factor which is often overlooked, although it is, of course, often accompanied by poor eating habits: if you're worried you may eat too quickly or forget to eat at all. Aspirin tablets, particularly the non-soluble variety, can also cause indigestion.

You can prevent the onset of indigestion, simply by avoiding the causes I've outlined.

It is important to visit a doctor if your indigestion pains persist for more than five days, if they recur regularly after fairly small and ordinarily digestible meals, or if they occur between meals or at night when you are asleep. Persistent or recurrent indigestion suggests the development of some sort of peptic ulceration and that needs to be properly investigated and treated. If your indigestion pains are accompanied by weight loss, persistent loss of appetite, or severe vomiting, then you need to see a doctor without delay. If the pains are severe or if the vomiting involves obvious blood or any dark brown material (old blood) then a doctor's immediate attention is needed.

It is fairly well known that you can avoid indigestion by avoiding certain foods, by eating small, regular meals, by nibbling between meals and by taking indigestion remedies regularly. If you do any of these things to avoid indigestion pains then you need your doctor's advice. Your indigestion may well involve some ulceration of the stomach or duodenum and that ulceration may require treatment rather than symptomatic relief.

It is the stomach's job to turn the vast variety of foodstuffs it receives into a movable thick soup. To facilitate this the cells of the stomach lining produce something like three litres of gastric juice a day. Gastric juice production is increased by stress, alcohol, hunger and nicotine. The most important constituent of the gastric juice is hydrochloric acid: an acid strong enough to burn holes in your carpet. It is that acid which helps to produce the pain associated with indigestion, gastritis and ulceration. And that is why indigestion remedies provide only symptomatic relief. They don't interfere with the production of excess acid or have any effect on the stomach lining – they simply neutralize some of the acid.

Most popular indigestion remedies consist of nothing more or less than antacids. Proprietary medicines are often available as liquids, powders and tablets. Liquids and powders usually work better than tablets, which need to be sucked or chewed thoroughly before being swallowed, but it is obviously easier to carry tablets around in your pocket or handbag than it is to carry a huge bottle of medicine! If you do suffer from occasional, mild attacks of indigestion it is probably best to keep tablets with you or in the car and a bottle of medicine in the home medicine cupboard.

There are a great many antacids available and no one is obviously superior. Each compound has its disadvantages, producing side effects which affect different people in different ways. It is to overcome these side effects that manufacturers mix together two or more antacids in their medicines, although since side effects usually take a day or two to appear, while indigestion is for most people a fleeting problem, cheaper, non-branded versions are usually quite suitable.

Sodium bicarbonate is one of the best-known and most easily available antacids. This is found in baking soda, which is a useful temporary stand-by, and although it isn't suitable for long-term treatment (because of the side effects it can have) it can be used to provide relief on a Saturday evening when the chemists' shops are all shut.

Most of the other products which are sold contain aluminium, magnesium or calcium compounds. All of these compounds have their own particular problems and may therefore be suitable for one sufferer but not for another. Magnesium compounds, for example, tend to have a laxative effect and are, therefore, suitable for people who tend to be rather constipated. Aluminium compounds tend to have a constipating effect and so they are more useful for people whose bowels tend to be 'on the loose side'. For a non-branded antacid choose from *Aluminium Hydroxide Tablets BP, Magnesium Hydroxide Mixture BP* or *Magnesium Trisilicate Mixture BPC*. Non-branded mixtures are also available as *Compound Calcium Carbonate Powder BPC* (which contains calcium carbonate, sodium bicarbonate and magnesium carbonate) and *Compound Magnesium Trisilicate Tablets BPC* (which contain magnesium trisilicate and aluminium hydroxide).

These five products are likely to be as effective as many of the much more expensive, widely advertised brands.

Branded preparations which contain one or more of aluminium hydroxide, calcium carbonate or magnesium trisilicate as major ingredients, and which should all be effective, include *Alka-Mints*, *Aludrox, Birley's Antacid Powder, Boots Dyspepsia Tablets, Boots Indigestion Tablets, De Witt's Antacid Powder, De Witt's Antacid Tablets, Dijex, Droxalin Tablets, Eso-Dex Indigestion Tablets, Gastrils, Gaviscon, Gelusil, Indi-Go, Maalox, Macleans Indigestion Powder, Macleans Indigestion Tablets, Moorland Indigestion Tablets, Nulacin, Primes Premiums, Rhuaka Indigestion Tablets, Setlers, Titralac* and *Tums*.

Apart from these three compounds there are a large number of other aluminium, calcium and magnesium compounds used in the manufacture of antacids. Aluminium phosphate, magnesium carbonate and magnesium hydroxide are commonly used.

Magnesium hydroxide is the basic ingredient of *Boots Cream of Magnesia Tablets* and the big-selling *Milk of Magnesia* (tablets and liquid). *Mil-Par* contains magnesium hydroxide together with liquid paraffin (see p.88). *Rennie Digestif Tablets,* another big-selling antacid, contain chalk and magnesium carbonate.

Abdine, Abdine Double Strength, Bablets, Boots Alkaline Stomach Powder, Boots Indigestion Mixture, Cox's Digestive Mints, Dolomite Tablets, Meggeson Dyspepsia Tablets, Opas Indigestion Powder and Tablets, Rodale and *Ventos Stomach Powder* all contain magnesium, sodium, calcium or aluminium compounds. Again, these products should all help.

Whatever antacid is selected it should be taken in relatively large doses, quite frequently. The maximum dose recommended by the manufacturers may need to be taken every two hours. With non-branded products I suggest doses as follows: *Aluminium Hydroxide Tablets BP* – 1 or 2 tablets; *Compound Calcium Carbonate Powder BPC* – up to 5 gm; *Magnesium Hydroxide Mixture BP* – 10 ml; *Magnesium Trisilicate Mixture BPC* – 20 ml. Once relief has been obtained the medicine can be stopped or the dosage at least reduced.

Children with indigestion should be given a small amount of warm milk and possibly a small dose of an adult antacid mixture.

Some antacid mixtures also include dimethicone (also known as dimethylpolysiloxane) which helps gases in the stomach escape. It does this by helping small bubbles of air coalesce to form larger bubbles.

The following compounds are therefore particularly suitable for people who have wind they cannot expel: *Andursil, Antasil, Asilone, Diloran, Polycrol Gel, Polycrol Tablets, Siloxyl, Sovol Liquid* and *Sovol Tablets*.

The final antacid mixture to be mentioned is *Alka Seltzer*, a unique and, to some people, surprising combination of sodium bicarbonate and aspirin. This famous, big-selling compound is used in the treatment of headaches and indigestion and is particularly recommended for 'headache with upset stomach' – the sort of thing you get if you eat or drink too much the night before. The manufacturers have collected a great deal of evidence which shows that this combination is not as dangerous to people with stomach troubles as it might seem to be. Nevertheless, despite their reassurances I find it difficult to recommend this product.

Apart from the antacids I have already mentioned there are other substances used in the treatment of indigestion. Liquorice has long been used in herbal mixtures and is today available in *Rabro* and *Caved-S* (which, just for good measure, also contains bismuth subnitrate, aluminium hydroxide, magnesium carbonate and sodium bicarbonate). Charcoal is another long-established remedy which is available as a powder, granule, tablet or biscuit and which is said to help absorb gases. Products which contain charcoal include *Bragg's Charcoal Biscuits, Bragg's Charcoal Tablets, Carbomucil, Charabs, Darco G-60, Eucarbon, Golden Health Indigestion Tablets, Lustys Charcoal Tablets, Potter's Acidosis Tablets,* and if your dog gets indigestion, *Bragg's Charcoal Dog Biscuits*.

However, the value of charcoal as an indigestion remedy is, in my opinion, doubtful.

A number of bismuth salts are used in the treatment of indigestion. Bismuth is supposed to have an antacid and protective action, but these effects have not been proven. Bismuth compounds used include bismuth carbonate, bismuth hydroxide, bismuth salicylate, acid bismuth sodium tartrate, bismuth subnitrate, bismuth aluminate and bismuth and ammonium citrate.

Proprietary preparations which include bismuth (as well as other antacids) are *Ayrtons Heart Shape Indigestion Tablets, Bisma-Calna Cream, Bismag Powder, Bisma-Rex Antacid Tablets, BiSoDol Powder, BiSoDol Tablets, BM Indigestion Suspension, Boots Frangula Compound Tablets, Ovals Indigestion Tablets* and *Roter Tablets*. It is difficult to choose between the antacid products I have listed in this section, but the standard non-branded preparations are probably cheaper than most and just as effective.

There are inevitably a number of herbal remedies available. These include *Biobalm, Box's Indigestion Pills, Heath and Heather's Indigestion and Flatulence Tablets, Heath and Heather's Indigestion Tablets, Potter's D4 Special Formula Stomach Tablets* and *Thompsons Indigestion Remedy*. *Biobalm* is also sometimes recommended for thickening soups, gravies and sauces. I make no further comment.

Health salts are sometimes used by sufferers in the treatment of upset stomachs, but I feel that other products I have mentioned are likely to be more suitable.

MENSTRUATION

There are a number of products available for use by women who experience pain during their monthly periods.

The symptoms of premenstrual tension vary a good deal. In the past most of the treatments offered have been designed to deal with specific symptoms (such as headaches, ankle swelling, and so on). Recently, research has shown that there are real physical causes for premenstrual tension which may be cured (temporarily or permanently) by the use of vitamin B6 (pyridoxine), see p.180.

My advice to a woman who suffers from premenstrual tension and who would like to try treatment with pyridoxine would be to visit her own doctor first. There are, after all, other possible treatments which are not available without a prescription and which might prove suitable.

Those women who genuinely find it impossible to obtain pyridoxine on prescription can, however, purchase vitamin B6 tablets themselves. A dosage of 20–40 mg twice a day (totalling 40–80 mg) seems to help many women. The tablets should be taken for three days before symptoms are expected, during the time that symptoms appear or usually appear, and for three days after the disappearance of symptoms. Vitamin B6 is excreted from the body if taken in excess so potential risks are small, although some women find that even fairly low doses cause indigestion-type symptoms. After six months the vitamin tablets may be left off for a while and if symptoms recur then they can be taken again.

Incidentally, although the symptoms of premenstrual tension vary enormously from woman to woman there is one crucial diagnostic pointer: premenstrual tension problems *always* occur before a period and at approximately the same time in a sufferer's cycle.

Women whose main complaint is of fluid retention are recommended by the advertisers to take a product called *Aqua Ban.* I do not recommend any diuretic (see p.51).

Tampax are probably the best-known makers of tampons. Their name has gone into the language together with Hoover and Biro. They and *Lil-lets*, among others, make a range of tampons.

Towels are made by a considerable number of manufacturers. Well-known brands include *Dr White's, Kotex Simplicity, Kotex Sylphs, Libra* and *Lilia,* and brands designed for use by women whose inter-menstrual discharge is noticeable include *Carefree Panty Shields* and *Kotex Brevia.*

MIGRAINE (see also **Pain** p.134)

Millions of working days are lost each year through migraine. The sufferers are said to have included Lewis Carroll, Darwin, Freud, Joan of Arc, Rudyard Kipling, Nietzsche and Jefferson. It has been said that 10% of the population have migraine attacks from time to time. The symptoms vary a great deal but, in addition to a searing headache, many patients vomit. Before the headache there may also be a warning 'aura'. Some sufferers see flashing lights and visual disturbances are common. Migraines usually begin in the sufferer's teens and may persist throughout the victim's life. They occur at irregular intervals, sometimes once or twice a week, usually less frequently.

The cause of migraine is still something of a mystery, but it seems likely that the blood vessels supplying the brain constrict and then dilate, reducing and then increasing the flow of blood to the brain. The initial constriction causes the aura, the following dilation produces the pain. In tension headache the pain is caused by too much blood flowing into the brain. The same thing happens in high blood pressure. In migraine it is often the blood vessels on one side of the head that are affected; hence the result that the headache occurs on one side of the head.

Migraine attacks are 'triggered' off by many different things. Sometimes a specific factor can be found which causes the attacks. Chocolate, cheese, oranges, lemons, shellfish, alcohol, tobacco, bananas and fried foods have been described as causing migraine attacks. To find out whether or not any of these 'triggers' is responsible a migraine sufferer must keep a close record of all he or she consumes for a month or two. Only then may a pattern showing some relationship between migraine attacks and a foodstuff be discovered. Making lists may be tiresome but it does frequently help pinpoint a cause.

When migraine attacks are caused by stress they usually occur when the subject is relaxing, and often at weekends. Any form of excitement may produce the telltale symptoms of a migraine attack and pleasure as well as unhappiness can produce the pain.

When an attack occurs the pain and discomfort may be relieved by ordinary painkillers but often something more powerful is needed. The classic treatment is a drug called ergotamine tartrate which helps by constricting the dilated arteries supplying the brain. The ergotamine does not, however, help relieve the visual symptoms. Other drugs are said to help by reducing the responsiveness of the cranial arteries.

Migraleve is one of the best-known products used in the treatment of migraine and available without a prescription. There are pink and yellow tablets. The pink ones contain buclizine dihydrochloride (an antihistamine), paracetamol, codeine phosphate and dioctylsodium sulphosuccinate (which is described on p.88, and which is presumably included to counteract the effects of the codeine). Two pink tablets are used at the first sign of an attack. Yellow *Migraleve* tablets, used at the rate of two every four hours if pain persists, consist of paracetamol, codeine phosphate and dioctylsodium sulphosuccinate.

There does not seem to me to be any great advantage in using these tablets as opposed to ordinary painkilling tablets. Many other products are available only on prescription and patients who suffer regularly from migraine attacks should consult a doctor.

MOUTH PROBLEMS
Mouth ulcers or aphthous ulcers are found under the tongue, on the inner side of the lower lip, or on the inner side of the cheeks. At least that is where they are most commonly found; they can be found anywhere in the mouth. Although they are extremely small and may indeed

be hardly visible, they cause a great deal of pain. They are white, rarely more than a couple of millimetres across and last on average for a week or ten days. They often occur in groups of three or four.

No one really knows what causes them but the unfortunate folk who suffer tend to keep on suffering. The only optimistic note is that as the years go by they usually occur less frequently.

Physical trauma (slipping with the toothbrush or chewing something particularly hard) can cause aphthous ulcers but the most important cause seems to be stress. Some people get indigestion when under stress, some get headaches and others get aphthous ulcers. There are a number of treatments around which are designed to provide symptomatic relief: there is no cure as yet.

Among the leading products are *Rinstead Pastilles* and *Rinstead Gel*. The pastilles are said to sell approximately 30 million packs a year and consist of a mixture of antiseptics and ingredients intended to relieve pain. They do seem to provide an acceptable amount of relief. *Rinstead Gel* contains benzocaine (an anaesthetic) which is also an ingredient of *Cox's Mouth Ulcer Lozenges, Cupal Mouth Ulcer Tablets* and *Ora-jel*. *Anbesol, Medijel, Medijel Pastilles* and *Mulcets Gel* all contain another anaesthetic – lignocaine. *Oralcer* contains clioquinol (see p.110) and I do not recommend it. *Mulcets Mouth Ulcer Tablets* contain ascorbic acid (vitamin C) and cetylpyridinium chloride which is an antiseptic. I think that products containing benzocaine or lignocaine should provide useful relief.

Mouthwashes and gargles are advertised as being suitable for a wide range of conditions including mouth ulcers, sore throats, gum infections and soreness. The following products all contain at least one antiseptic or disinfectant: *Bansor Mouth and Throat Antiseptic, Betadine Gargle and Mouthwash, Boots Antiseptic Mouthwash and Gargle, Dentosine* and *Listerine Antiseptic*. There are also a number of gels, lotions and pastilles designed to help relieve soreness of the gums. These include *Gum-eze, Smith's Red Gum and Menthol Pastilles, Tellora D3, Three Flasks Sore Gum Lotion* and *Tyordac Gum Pastilles*. Most minor mouth infections will clear up by themselves and more serious infections need the attention of a dentist or doctor. *Corsodyl* (available as a gel or mouthwash) which is recommended in the treatment of gingivitis (gum infection and inflammation) has been reported to stain the teeth.

Cold sores, like mouth ulcers, are small, painful and common.

Menthol and camphor are both said to have a soothing effect. One or both of these substances are available in the following products: *Ayrtons Cold Sore Lotion, Boots Cold Sore Lotion, Cold Sore Lotion, Candol Cold Sore Salve, Cupal Cold Sore Cream* and *Three Flasks Cold Sore Lotion.* Dryness and soreness of the lips caused by an allergy to a cosmetic, or by sun or wind, can be eased by using zinc and castor oil cream or calamine cream or any suitable plain cream. *Zinc and Castor Oil Ointment BP* and *Calamine Ointment BPC* are non-branded substances which are useful. These are probably as helpful and effective as commercial, branded products.

MUSCULAR ACHES AND PAINS

The simplest, cheapest and most effective treatment for any muscular ache (presuming that the muscle has not been torn or damaged and does not need any sort of physical support) is aspirin. There are products which are specifically advertised for the treatment of rheumatic pains but which contain aspirin. *Cojene, Fynnon Calcium Aspirin* and *30 Days Rheumatic Tablets* are but three of the aspirin-based products recommended by their manufacturers for the relief of rheumatic pains. In my opinion these are no better than other forms of aspirin described on p.134.

More popular than aspirin but probably less effective are the rheumatic balms, ointments, embrocations and rubbing liniments which are available. These work in several ways: they may irritate the skin thereby distracting the patient from the deep muscular pains, they may simply smell good and have a placebo effect, or they may help because they provide a good excuse for some gentle massage. It is certainly true that rubbing an affected part of the body can do wonders, and rubbing oils do make massaging easier to perform. Those liniments which irritate the skin dilate superficial blood vessels and therefore produce redness and warmth. Similar effects can be obtained by applying heat to the muscles either through a hot-water bottle (see p.141) or a warm bath. The heat increases the circulation in the skin and also deeper in the tissues.

It is important to remember that rubbing oils and other substances should not be used on cracked, cut or infected skin.

Choosing a liniment or balm, rub or embrocation is largely a matter of taste, or rather smell. I don't feel that there is a great deal to choose between the following products on purely medical grounds: *Algesal, Algipan, Aradolene, Aspellin, Atlas Athletic Embrocation, Balmosa, Bayolin, Bengue's Balsam, Boots Embrocation, Boots Menthol and Wintergreen Embrocation, Boots Pain Relieving Balm, Buxton Rubbing Bottle, Cremalgex, Cremalgin, Cremathurm R, Deep Heat, Eade's Anodyne Rheumatic Balm, Elliman's Embrocation, Embrolin, Fibrosine Balm, Fiery Jack Rubbing Cream, Fisherman's Friend Rubbing Ointment, Garlisol Rheumatic Balm, George's American Marvel Liniment, Glenol Rubbing Oils, Goddard's White Oil Embrocation, Gonne Analgesic Cream, Infurno Embrocation, Infurno Massage Cream, Intralgin, Kil-pain Menthol and Wintergreen Cream with Mustard, Menthol and Wintergreen Cream, Mentholatum Balm, Mentholatum Deep Heat Rub, Nasciodine Medicated Massage Cream, Panigo Balm, Parkinsons White Embrocation, Radian A Spirit Dressing, Radian B Spirit Liniment, Radian Massage Cream, Ralgex Balm, Ralgex Embrocation Stick, Samaritan Menthol and Wintergreen Cream, Seven Rubbing Oils, Sloan's Liniment, Soothene Ointment, Tiger Balm, Transvasin* and *Vadarex Wintergreen Ointment. Algipan* and *Deep Heat* are among the most popular of these remedies.

Choosing a rub (the words balm, embrocation, rub and liniment are interchangeable for all practical purposes) can be done on a price and weight basis. *Compound Methyl Salicylate Ointment BPC* (oil of wintergreen) is a relatively cheap non-branded rub. Many of the branded rubs contain methyl salicylate as an important ingredient. Since this substance has the actions of aspirin but is well absorbed through the skin it can have a direct effect on the troubled muscles.

Witch hazel, often used for cooling and soothing bruises and sprains, is another ingredient of branded products and can be bought as *Witch Hazel BPC. Turpentine Liniment BP* and *White Liniment BPC* are also available and effective.

It is fashionable today to put everything into spray cans. So there are sprays available for use on aching muscles. These are often used with miraculous effect on wounded footballers! Products in this category include *Aerocol Pain Relieving Spray, Dubam, PR Spray, Ralgex Analgesic Spray* and *Skefron.* Bath salts which are designed to help people with muscular ailments include, among others, *Luma Medicated Bath Salts, Radian Bath Salts* and *Radox.* Hot baths, with or without added ingredients, will almost certainly provide some relief.

Copper bracelets and bangles have long been popular but there is no scientific evidence that I know of which shows that these are more effective than other old wives' cures. Those fascinated by the unusual may be interested to know that the following have been recommended for the prevention of rheumatism: carrying the right foot of a hare in the left pocket; putting a nutmeg, mole's paw, piece of brimstone, female hedgehog jaw, potato, magnet or cork in any pocket; swallowing a spider or carrying one round in a small box; and making a necklace out of chestnuts gathered by rheumatism-free children. Sufferers seeking a solution have been advised to eat celery, drink poppy tea, tie an adder's skin around the leg, thrash affected parts of the body with stinging nettles, drink tea made from willow bark, or arrange to be stung by bees. Drinking tea made from willow bark is particularly interesting since it was from the willow tree that aspirin was first isolated.

There are an enormous number of herbal remedies available for the treatment of rheumatic and other muscular ailments. I know of no evidence suggesting that any of them are more effective than ordinary aspirin tablets. Nor is there any evidence that convinces me that electrical massagers are more effective than ordinary hand massage. They are certainly more expensive. I do not recommend enzyme preparations such as *Chymoral* for the home treatment of muscular or soft tissue disorders.

One of the best-known remedies for rheumatic pains is *Fynnon Salt*. The main ingredient of this product is sodium sulphate which is a laxative. There is no medical evidence that I know of which supports the use of laxatives in the treatment of muscular aches and pains or any form of rheumatism. Other health salts which are described on pp.89-90 also contain laxatives.

Any muscular ache or pain which does not improve after five days' treatment with aspirin or paracetamol tablets, or which is not relieved by massage within a similar period of time, should be treated by a doctor. Muscular damage resulting from injury may need to be examined by a doctor without home remedies being applied. Any pain, swelling or limitation of movement which deteriorates rather than improves after treatment should be treated professionally.

PAIN

Pain is a symptom your body uses to tell you when there is something wrong. Primarily it is a defence mechanism. If you sit on a pin you'll jump up; if you burn your hand you'll pull it away.

Painkillers (or analgesics) will alleviate the symptom but they will not usually affect the cause. It is important to remember this for two reasons. Firstly, although you may feel better after having taken a painkiller your body may still need to be used with caution; strained muscles can be permanently damaged if overstretched because the normal constraints afforded by pain mechanisms have been over-ruled. Secondly, if you need to keep taking painkillers then you need to see a doctor. Painkillers should never be taken indefinitely. The five-day rule should be applied. This section deals only with painkillers for oral use. Liniments and rubs are dealt with on p.131.

Specific pains

Specific pains are dealt with elsewhere in this book as follows:

Backache (p.68)
Earache (p.112)
Headache (p.120)
Migraine (p.128)
Muscle and joint pains (p.131)
Period pains (p.142)
Toothache (p.176)

Aspirin

Although the effectiveness of salicylic acid was described in a scientific paper over 200 years ago it was not until the end of the nineteenth century that aspirin tablets came on to the market and were readily obtainable from chemists' shops. The growth of this drug in the last three-quarters of a century has been phenomenal.

Today aspirin is widely recognized as a painkiller, an antipyretic (a drug that brings down the patient's temperature) and an anti-inflammatory drug (a drug which reduces the sort of inflammation that occurs in muscles and joints in rheumatism and arthritis).

It is effective against all forms of mild to moderate pain. We still do not really know how it works.

Paracetamol

Paracetamol is the other main ingredient of popular home painkillers. It is chemically similar to phenacetin, a drug which is now very much out of favour in view of its toxic effects on the kidneys. Paracetamol has antipyretic and painkilling qualities similar to those of aspirin. Its properties are not as well documented as those of aspirin, but because of the publicity which has been given to the effects aspirin can have on the stomach paracetamol is rapidly gaining in popularity.

The hazards of aspirin

The hazards and risks of taking aspirin have perhaps been too well documented. In fact, considering the number of aspirin tablets which are taken annually (aspirin is the world's No. 1 drug and 2000 tons of aspirin are swallowed in Britain every year) the side effects associated with the drug are relatively slight but have been overemphasized by companies with alternative and allegedly superior products on the market.

The main potential problems are, of course, stomach discomfort, heartburn and bleeding. If you experience any stomach upset after taking aspirin, or if you have a history of any stomach disorder, then you would probably be wise to choose paracetamol instead. Aspirin is not suitable as a treatment for stomach disorders or indigestion, although the manufacturers of *Alka Seltzer* claim that their particular product is safe because of its special composition.

If the dose of aspirin taken is too high you may suffer from dizziness, headache or ringing in the ears. These symptoms do not necessarily mean that you should stop taking aspirin but that you should reduce the dosage.

Anyone suspected of having taken an overdose of aspirin tablets should be seen in hospital as soon as possible. 25–30 gm of aspirin can be lethal but people have recovered after having swallowed three times as much as this.

The hazards of paracetamol

Side effects and problems are uncommon with paracetamol but overdosage of paracetamol can cause serious liver damage. Anyone who is suspected of having taken an overdose of paracetamol should be seen at a hospital urgently even if there do not appear to be any symptoms.

Aspirin or paracetamol?

These two drugs are the most common constituents of painkilling tablets and medicines. They are, to a large extent, interchangeable although, naturally, people who suffer from uncomfortable, painful or threatening side effects after taking one product will use another.

Both have similar qualities in reducing fevers but aspirin is probably a slightly better painkiller than paracetamol. The main advantage which paracetamol has is that it is available as a liquid as well as a tablet.

Selection is largely a matter of personal choice but if you don't mind which you use aspirin is probably the better buy. If you can't take aspirin or don't like swallowing tablets then use paracetamol liquid.

How to take aspirin

Aspirin is most effective and safest if taken with milk or water after food. It works most effectively when taken with *warm* water. Soluble aspirin works quicker than the non-soluble variety.

How to take paracetamol

Paracetamol should be taken with water on an empty stomach but it can be taken after food.

Non-branded aspirin and paracetamol

Non-branded painkillers control pain just as well as extensively and expensively advertised products.

Aspirin is available as *Aspirin Tablets BP* and *Soluble Aspirin Tablets BP*. The former are available as 300 mg tablets and the latter usually contain 300 mg of aspirin together with citric acid, calcium carbonate and saccharin. In practice up to twelve 300 mg tablets of ordinary aspirin can be taken by adults over a 24 hour period. The dosage of *Soluble Aspirin Tablets BP* for children between the ages of six and twelve should be one tablet up to four times a day. *Paediatric Soluble*

Aspirin Tablets BPC contain 75 mg of aspirin and the recommended doses are:

age **dose**
1–2 1–2 up to 4 times a day
3–5 3–4 up to 3 times a day
6–12 4 up to 4 times a day

Paracetamol is available as *Paracetamol Tablets BP* in 500 mg tablets. The dosage should be up to a maximum of 1000 mg four times a day. *Paediatric Paracetamol Elixir BPC* contains 120 mg of paracetamol in 5 ml and can be given as a single 5 ml dose to infants under one year of age and in double doses to children over one year.

Non-branded mixtures are also available. There are *Aspirin and Caffeine Tablets BP*, *Aspirin and Codeine Tablets BP* and *Soluble Aspirin and Codeine Tablets BP*.

In my opinion no branded analgesics have any important advantages over these compounds.

Variations on the aspirin theme
Apart from ordinary, common or garden aspirin tablets there are many variations on this well-established theme. Soluble aspirin tablets (such as *Soluble Aspirin Tablets BP*) contain aspirin together with calcium carbonate and citric acid and can be dissolved in water before being taken. Soluble aspirin is more rapidly absorbed than standard aspirin but whether or not it causes less side effects seems uncertain.

Buffered aspirin tablets contain drugs which affect the pH of the stomach contents and reduce the risk of the stomach wall being injured. Some buffered products are fizzy or effervescent because they contain sodium bicarbonate and citric acid (*Alka Seltzer* and *Clarapin* fall into this category).

There are some brands of aspirin (*Nu-Seals*) which are enteric-coated – that is they are protected by a relatively insoluble coating which allows the delayed release of the aspirin in the small intestine – and there are other brands which consist of minute aspirin particles bound together and designed to be released slowly in the stomach (*Levius*, for example).

Aspirin is sometimes combined with aluminium (as in *Palaprin Forte*) and it is available in a specially prepared suspension (*Benoral*), as a chewable preparation (*Aspergum*), see p.82, and coated with paracetamol (*Safapryn*).

There are even different formulations of the ordinary standard aspirin tablet and manufacturers sometimes claim that their product is put together in such a way that it falls apart more speedily, more safely or more efficiently than anyone else's standard aspirin tablet. These claims should probably be taken with a pinch of salt, a dash of quinine and a few micrograms of whatever else your hand falls on in the laboratory.

Despite all the research work which has been done there is no evidence that I know of which shows that any of these preparations are more effective, or safer than plain *Soluble Aspirin Tablets BP* for ordinary use. This product has the added advantage that it is probably the cheapest way to buy soluble aspirin.

Variations on the paracetamol theme

There are fewer variations on the tablet or liquid form of paracetamol, but an effervescent tablet (*Para Seltzer*) is available which also contains a small quantity of caffeine. *Panadol Soluble* is also effervescent but it does not contain any caffeine.

Brands of aspirin

The following branded home medicines contain aspirin or an aspirin alternative as the analgesic. The amount of actual aspirin contained in each tablet is listed in milligrams after each name: *Alka Seltzer* (324 mg), *Anadin* (325 mg), *Angiers Junior Aspirin* (81 mg), *Aspergum* (227 mg), *Aspro* (324 mg), *Aspro Clear* (300 mg), *Beechams Powders* (540 mg), *Beechams Powder Tablets* (270 mg), *Boots Children's Soluble Aspirin* (75 mg), *Caprin* (324 mg), *Cephos Powders* (570 mg), *Cephos Tablets* (285 mg), *Claradin* (300 mg), *Cox's Junior Soluble Aspirin* (75 mg), *Disprin* (300 mg), *Disprin Junior* (81 mg), *Effervescent Aspro* (300 mg), *Fennings' Soluble Junior Aspirin* (75 mg), *Fynnon Calcium Aspirin* (500 mg), *Genasprin* (300 mg), *Grovisprin* (300 mg), *Laboprin* (300 mg), *Levius* (500 mg), *Miniprins Soluble Aspirin Tablets for Children* (75 mg), *Nu-Seals Aspirin* (300 mg and 600 mg), *Phensic* (325 mg) and *Solprin* (300 mg).

Brands of paracetamol

The following branded home medicines contain paracetamol as the only painkilling ingredient. The amount of paracetamol in each tablet or 5 ml of syrup is listed in milligrams after the name: *Baxen Tablets* (250 mg), *Benzac Tablets* (250 mg), *Calpol* (120 mg), *Child's Pain Elixir* (120 mg), *Codural Period Pain Tablets* (250 mg), *Eso-Pax Capsules* (240 mg), *Femerital* (250 mg), *Fennings' Adult Cooling Powders* (180 mg), *Fennings' Soluble Children's Cooling Tablets* (30 mg), *Flu-rex* (400 mg), *Hedex* (500 mg), *Hedex Seltzer* (1 gm), *Hush* (120 mg), *Panaleve Elixir* (120 mg), *Panaleve Tablets* (500 mg), *Panadol* (500 mg), *Panasorb* (500 mg), *Panets* (500 mg), *Panets Baby Syrup* (120 mg), *Para Seltzer* (500 mg), *Pirisol Junior Pain Tablets* (100 mg), *Placidex* (120 mg) and *PP Tablets* (150 mg).

Other painkillers

Aloxiprin is a chemical combination of aluminium oxide and aspirin and it has very similar properties to aspirin. It is, however, said to be less likely to cause stomach upsets than aspirin and could therefore be of use to those who are unable to take aspirin tablets because of gastric side effects. Aloxiprin is available as *Palaprin Forte*, each tablet of which is approximately equivalent to 500 mg of aspirin.

Acetyl salicylic acid, acid acetylsal and acidum acetylsalicylicum are all pseudonyms for aspirin.

Salicylamide is similar to aspirin for all practical purposes.

Codeine is an effective analgesic but cannot be bought without a prescription in an effective dose. It can cause constipation and is addictive.

Analgesic mixtures

There are a great many composite pain-relieving tablets available for use at home. The three commonest constituents are aspirin, paracetamol and codeine.

Tablets which contain aspirin (or an aspirin type of drug) and paracetamol include *Actron, Chilvax Tablets, De Witt's Analgesic Pills* (which in fact contain lithium salicylate rather than ordinary aspirin and which I do not recommend), *Doan's Backache Pills, Nurse Sykes Powders, Nurse Sykes Tablets, Persomnia, Powerin, PR Tablets, Restwell* and *Safapryn.*

The following products contain aspirin and codeine phosphate: *Codis, Cojene* and *Paxedin Tablets.*

There are also products which contain paracetamol and codeine phosphate: *Cox's Pain Relief Tablets, EP Tablets, Panadeine Co, Pandrin, Paracodol* and *Parahypon.*

Finally there is *Veganin* which contains all three analgesics.

I do not believe that there is any advantage in using a painkiller which contains a mixture of two, three or more painkillers.

The added ingredients
Painkilling tablets often contain drugs and chemicals which are not painkillers. If you've followed my advice and you begin to study bottle labels when shopping for home medicines you'll undoubtedly come across some of the following constituents: caffeine, calcium carbonate, calcium phosphate, citric acid (which may or may not be described as anhydrous), magnesium carbonate, quinine, saccharin and sodium bicarbonate.

Caffeine is included in the belief that since pain and tiredness often go together the stimulation provided by caffeine will be welcome. The fact is that in many preparations there is less caffeine than there is in a cup of coffee. Anyway I do not think that it is good pharmaceutical practice to mix drugs unless you really have to. The more constituents there are in a product the greater are the chances of side effects and allergic reactions occurring. In addition there is also a risk of constituent chemicals reacting together to produce unexpected effects. The safest products are usually the simplest.

The properties of caffeine are described in greater detail on p.174. The following home medicines include caffeine: *Actron, Anadin, Askit Powders, Askit Tablets, Baxen Tablets, Beechams Powders, Beechams Powders Tablets, Benzac Tablets, Cal-mo Rheumatic Tablets, Cephos Powders, Cephos Tablets, Chilvax Tablets, Codural Period Pain Tablets, Cojene, Cox's Pain*

Relief Tablets, EP Tablets, Eso-Pax Capsules, Fennings' Adult Cooling Powders, Flu-rex, Hedex Seltzer, Mrs Cullen's Powders, Nurse Sykes Powders, Nurse Sykes Tablets, Pandrin, Phensic, Powerin, PP Tablets, PR Tablets and *Yeast-Vite*.

Calcium carbonate and calcium phosphate, magnesium carbonate and sodium bicarbonate are all antacids which are there to counteract the effect of the powerful acid floating around in your stomach.

Citric acid is there to make the whole thing fizz nicely.

Quinine and saccharin are probably included for flavouring as much as anything else although in larger doses quinine has a number of medicinal uses.

Finally, there are a number of products which contain various other unique mixtures. *Askit Powders* and *Askit Tablets* contain aspirin, aloxiprin and aluminium glycinate as well as caffeine. Aloxiprin is a product with similar actions to aspirin and aluminium glycinate is an antacid. *Togal Tablets* contain aspirin and lithium citrate together with quinine dihydrochloride. Quinine dihydrochloride has mild analgesic properties but is most useful in the treatment of malaria while lithium citrate is today used for the treatment of manic-depression. *Cal-mo Rheumatic Tablets* contain 160 mg of aspirin, caffeine and a minute quantity of phenylsemicarbazide, which is another painkiller and antipyretic. *Yeast-Vite*, which are advertised for headaches and tension, contain salicylamide, caffeine, clove, dried yeast and elements of vitamin B.

The hot-water bottle

The good old hot-water bottle should not be ignored as a pain reliever. Pain almost anywhere in the body can be eased by the judicious application of a hot-water bottle. To avoid burning the skin wrap the hot-water bottle in a thin towel or pillowcase or buy a cloth or knitted cover. Try to resist the temptation to buy bottles made in the shapes of animals – they may look cuddly, but they are not as safe.

A few words of warning: don't ever use a hot-water bottle that shows *any* signs of perishing. Make sure the screw top is well fitting and tightly fastened, exclude the air before you fasten the top and don't overfill the bottle.

Finally, remember that for sprains, bruises and strains a hot-water bottle can be filled with ice and cold water. It is not as messy as a compress, but it may be just as effective.

When to call a doctor

Any pain which is not eased or relieved after forty-eight hours needs to be diagnosed and treated by a doctor. Painkillers should never be taken for more than five consecutive days unless they have been prescribed by a doctor.

PERIOD PAINS (see also **Pain** p.134)

Period or menstrual pains are an important problem, affecting many millions of women every month and it has attracted the attention of many home medicine manufacturers. Among the 'specially formulated' products are *Feminax, Codural Period Pain Tablets* and *Femerital*.

Feminax contain paracetamol, salicylamide, codeine phosphate, caffeine and 100 micrograms of hyoscine hydrobromide. This latter substance, which is usually given in doses of 300–600 micrograms, has a number of qualities. It slows the heart, it calms excited patients and it induces sleep, it may prevent travel sickness and it is used as a pre-operative sedative. It is also used in the treatment of infantile cerebral palsy, paralysis agitans, and postencephalitic parkinsonism and is an antispasmodic.

Codural Period Pain Tablets contain paracetamol, caffeine and 1 mg of homatropine methylbromide which has properties not dissimilar to those associated with hyoscine hydrobromide. Homatropine methyl-bromide is usually given in doses of 2.5–5 mg.

Femerital contain an antispasmodic (ambucetamide) and paracetamol.

I suggest that initially the treatment of period pain be carried out in the same way as the treatment of any other sort of pain. Proprietary products can be tried if painkillers alone are of no use. If the pains are regularly too strong to be quelled by home medicines or if they are accompanied by heavy or unexpected bleeding then a doctor should be consulted.

PILES

Piles (or haemorrhoids) are simply varicose veins which occur around the anus. Although the cause isn't really known it is likely that they can be inherited and certain that chronic constipation, pregnancy and the excessive use of laxatives and purgatives can make them worse.

Itching, bleeding and a clear discharge are among the commonest early symptoms. Piles which can't be pushed back into the anal canal inevitably feel lumpy and uncomfortable and may be painful.

Before beginning to treat any of the symptoms which I have listed it is important to seek medical advice. More serious conditions can produce the same symptoms and even with the help of a bathroom mirror it isn't easy to make a precise diagnosis that is reliable. At the most try treatment for five days before asking for help.

There are a number of preparations available for easing and relieving the problems associated with piles. These are all intended to provide symptomatic relief rather than a cure.

Pills which are sold usually contain a laxative. *George's Pills for the Piles No. 3* and *Pile Tablets* both contain ingredients designed to ease constipation. Creams and ointments contain a variety of oils, antiseptics and other substances. They may soothe a little. The following products are widely available: *Anusol, Boots HP Ointment, Germoloids, Haemorex, Heath and Heather's Pile Ointment, ManZan Pile Ointment, Pilease, Pilogene, Preparation H* and *Pylatum Pile Ointment.* Some of these can be bought as both creams (or ointments) and suppositories. As is always the case with medicated creams patients who use some of these compounds may suffer allergic problems, particularly when the products are used for long periods of time. No treatment for piles should be used for more than five days without a doctor being consulted.

Inevitably, there are now sprays available for the treatment of piles – *Haemorrhoidal Spray* contains an antiseptic and an anaesthetic – and medicated wipes have also been introduced. I can see little point in spending money on these products.

To avoid suffering from piles it is important to avoid constipation. A diet which includes plenty of liquids and fruit and not too much carbohydrate will help. Once piles do develop discomfort can be relieved by putting bricks or books under the foot of the bed which helps the return of blood from the swollen veins to the heart, or by taking hot baths. Ice packs may also prove helpful.

PREGNANCY TESTS

In ancient Egypt women used to urinate on to the leaves of the papyrus plant. If the plant died they weren't pregnant, if it lived they were.

A general shortage of papyrus plants has led to the development of a number of less colourful ways of diagnosing pregnancy. Most of these depend on levels of specific hormones in the urine. There are two things to be remembered about all pregnancy tests: firstly, they cannot be used until a number of days after conception (the actual number of days depends on the test) and secondly, they may on occasion be wrong, producing both false positives and false negatives.

The best-known home test method is probably the *Predictor* test which can be used by a potential mother nine days after her period should have started. It seems simple to use. A few drops of urine are added to the test tube provided. The tube is then shaken and left for two hours. If the woman is pregnant a brown ring appears – if she isn't it doesn't. *Discover 2* is a similar test kit.

Almost every woman who has been pregnant will know that there are certain signs which tell her that she's expecting: she may feel sick, have enlarged, tender, tingling breasts and feel a need to pass urine more frequently than usual. A woman who has been pregnant in the past and who feels that she is pregnant again usually is.

Any woman who misses a period and does a pregnancy test which turns out negative should visit her doctor if she misses another period.

SICKNESS (vomiting)

There are many causes of sickness. Too much to eat or drink can cause a bout of vomiting as can the ingestion of infected food or drink. Such attacks of sickness may be followed by diarrhoea. There really isn't much you can do about this type of sickness except to drink large quantities of water (to replace the fluid that has been lost) and to make a mental note to avoid whatever it was you think may have caused the problem in the first place.

Anxiety or worry can cause vomiting. The phrase 'you make me sick' is well established in colloquial English. Gory, unpleasant sights may cause vomiting too. There isn't much that can be done to prevent this type of vomiting since it is usually unexpected and unpredictable.

Pregnancy is another common cause of sickness. Women are most commonly affected in the first few months of their pregnancy and the sickness usually (but not always) occurs in the mornings. Avoiding fatty smells, unpalatable foods and big meals may help, but if the sickness persists then a doctor's advice should be sought. There are pills you can buy without a prescription which will safely control the vomiting associated with pregnancy but I do not recommend pregnant women to take any medicines without medical advice.

The type of sickness that can best be helped with pills is motion sickness which is extremely common and very debilitating. Hippocrates wrote about motion sickness 2000 years ago, although he didn't divide it into car sickness, sea sickness, train sickness and plane sickness as we do now. He probably only had to deal with sea and chariot sickness.

A good deal of research has been done on the subject, much of it during and after the Second World War when high ranking army officers were struggling to find ways to stop sea sickness among soldiers being landed on enemy beaches. Field officers had discovered that soldiers are not at their best when as they've just dragged themselves from the landing craft.

Even more recently doctors involved in the American space programme have been studying the problems of motion sickness as it affects astronauts. Those doctors showed that a person who is nauseated by one type of motion isn't necessarily made ill by another. In other words a sailor who can get round the Horn without any problems at all may be dreadfully ill in an aeroplane.

Whatever the cause of the illness the symptoms usually follow a fairly reliable pattern. The patient will feel sweaty, sick and generally unwell. He'll probably be pale, he may salivate a good deal, and yawning seems to be a common symptom. Headaches and depression may follow and some sufferers just have to lie down and forget about the world for a while.

Depending on the conditions, between 10% and 100% of the people on a ship may develop sea sickness whereas the incidence of motion sickness on trains, planes and vehicles is much lower.

It isn't just the motion that causes the sickness. Other stimuli such as smells, noises and vibrations make things worse.

It is, incidentally, interesting that although children often suffer from motion sickness infants rarely do. Most of the children who suffer will grow out of it or will suffer less intensely.

One of the reasons for their 'growing out of it' is probably that they will become accustomed to the problem and they will adapt, learning how to suffer least. To help speed up that adaptation it is useful to help children by reassuring them when they feel ill and to divert their attention with a game or puzzle. The confidence which is acquired by successfully travelling without being sick will have an effect on future travelling.

Sickness sufferers can also help themselves by reclining or tilting their head back if they begin to feel ill. It's possible to do this in most planes, trains, cars or ships these days. And it is also a help to eat wisely before travelling. It is best to eat moderate amounts of fairly bland foods.

Just about everything that can be swallowed has been tried as an antidote to travel sickness. (I'm not going to discuss here all the 'magical' remedies such as putting brown paper down the back of a sufferer's shirt – except to refer you to the section on placebos (p.32) and to suggest that if the remedy works then it's a good one!) Antihistamines (see also p.50) have been found to be effective, and are the most commonly used drugs. They do unfortunately cause drowsiness and although this doesn't matter too much with children, it can be a disadvantage if it is the car driver who suffers from sickness.

Antihistamines which are available include cyclizine (sold as *Valoid*), dimenhydrinate (*Dramamine* and *Gravol*), meclozine (*Ancoloxin* and *Sea Legs*) and promethazine (*Avomine* and *Phenergan*). Of these, promethazine is probably one of the most effective. It may also be available as *Promethazine Elixir BPC* and *Promethazine Hydrochloride Tablets BP* but you will probably have to buy the named brands. I suggest one 25 mg tablet two hours before travelling for an adult and half a tablet for a child between six and twelve years. A 5 mg dose of promethazine as elixir can be given to a younger child if necessary. The dose can be given to adult or child the evening before travelling. Promethazine can also be used as a *treatment* for motion sickness. One tablet taken immediately and repeated at the following bedtime should suffice.

Anticholinergic drugs (see p.49) can also be used. They may produce a blurring of vision and should therefore be used with great caution by drivers. *Sereen* and *Quick Kwells* contain anticholinergics. *Joyrides* contain a smaller dose of an anticholinergic and are therefore recommended for children.

Sure Shield Adult Traveltabs contain chlorbutol, a mild sedative, which is probably less effective than the antihistamines and anti-cholinergics for the treatment of sea sickness.

SKIN DISORDERS
A number of skin problems are dealt with elsewhere in this book:

Acne (p.58)
Allergies (p.63)
Athlete's foot (p.117 and p.190)
Chilblains (p.70)
Corns and callouses (p.116)
Cuts and grazes (p.96)
Hair disorders (pp.105 and 118)
Ringworm (p.189)
Sunburn (p.161)
Sweating (p.166)

The value of vitamin creams and pills for skin troubles is discussed on p.180.

This section deals with more general skin problems and their solution. It is sometimes impossible and always difficult to differentiate between cosmetic skin products and medicinal ones. I have tried to omit references to cosmetics and cosmetic skin treatments, since the criteria for selection are obviously different to those relating to medicinal compounds. For example, creams, lotions and sprays which are advertised for the purpose of eradicating wrinkles, keeping the skin soft and young, reversing ageing processes and improving skin texture are not discussed; these are all cosmetic preparations and my feeling is that there is no point in my trying to discuss them in this book. What I have dealt with are the preparations designed to help in the treatment of skin disorders.

The commonest problem is probably simple dry skin. There are several causes for this. Long, leisurely hot baths can damage the skin and result in a loss of water and natural oils. Air conditioning and central heating also increase the loss of water from the skin. Too much sunbathing is also a possible cause of dry skin, although in the British climate this cause is probably relatively rare.

Preventing the development of dry skin by avoiding overlong soaks in the bath, by installing a humidifier or opening a window in the house or office, or by avoiding excessive exposure to the sun is obviously better than having to use creams in an attempt to repair and revitalize patches of dry skin. Incidentally, people with a tendency to develop dry skin may notice a deterioration after bathing in a chlorinated swimming pool: the chlorine may exacerbate dry skin problems.

Once dry skin has developed, however, ointments or oils are usually better than creams or soaps. Bath oils disperse in the bath water and adhere to the skin preventing the loss of natural water and oils. Alternatively, oil can be massaged into the skin after bathing. *Emulsifying Ointment BP* is a non-branded product which can be used. It is important to remember that ordinary toilet soap itself may make dry skin worse. *Aveeno Colloidal* and *Aveeno Oilated* are useful bath oils sometimes prescribed by doctors.

Another solution is to use an emollient regularly: these help to prevent loss of water from the surface of the skin and therefore help to re-hydrate the skin's surface layers. *E45 cream, Oilatum emollient, Ultrabase* and *Unguentum* are among the simple, branded products which are useful. These are likely to be considerably cheaper than and at least as effective as extremely expensive moisturizing creams and cosmetics, many of which simply contain added perfumes which contribute nothing to the effectiveness of the product, and do, in fact, increase the risk of allergic reactions developing.

It is sometimes forgotten that the human body can suffer bad effects from creams, ointments and other superficial treatments, just as it can from oral treatments.

There are a number of skin preparations which are designed to relieve itching and discomfort associated with dry skin conditions and with rashes, mild infections and other disorders. These may contain antihistamines (see p.50), calamine, zinc oxide or local anaesthetics such as benzocaine and lignocaine.

Calamine is a pink, insoluble powder which contains zinc carbonate and ferric oxide. It is sold in a number of different forms, being available in *Calsept, Cream of Calamine, Eczederm Cream, HEB Burn Cream, HEB Calamine* and *Lacto-Calamine Lotion* among others (see p.160). It is also available as *Calamine Lotion BP* and *Calamine Ointment BPC*. Calamine preparations help sooth and cool itchy, uncomfortable skin.

Zinc oxide is also soothing and protective and is available as *Compound Zinc Dusting Powder BPC, Zinc Cream BP* and *Zinc Ointment BP*. Many proprietary preparations for the treatment of nappy rash contain zinc oxide (see p.67).

Those skin preparations which include antiseptics and disinfectants should be avoided since they may cause irritation and are unlikely to help very much. Products containing local anaesthetics or antihistamines may be useful in the treatment of stings (see p.160) or allergic reactions (see p.63). Most other minor conditions can be eased with calamine or zinc oxide preparations. I do not recommend any home treatments intended specifically for the treatment of eczema, dermatitis or psoriasis. Any skin disorder which does not show signs of improvement after five days should be seen by a doctor and any skin blemish which gets bigger, bleeds, changes colour, ulcerates or hurts should be examined without delay.

Finally, there are available creams which can be used for the treatment of cracked skin and for protecting skin against exposure to irritants. Creams which contain silicone (such as *Atrixo* and *Vasogen*) and soft paraffin products (such as *Vaseline*) can be used to build a protective barrier for the skin.

SLEEPLESSNESS

It is while you are asleep that your brain recovers from the pressures and disasters of the day. While you're awake millions of pieces of information are fed into your brain every hour. Much of the information you are not even aware of is dealt with by your subconscious. During the hours in bed your batteries are recharged – and you should wake up ready for another few million bits and pieces of information.

The amount of sleep one individual needs may be very different to the amount needed by another. A newborn baby can need fifteen hours a day, and while one adult may happily get by with five hours a night another may become tired, irritable and depressed without nine hours' sleep. It's unfair, I know, but then who said anything about life being fair? Some people live to be a hundred while others don't even get into double figures.

But one fact doesn't vary: we all need some sleep. And if you aren't getting enough then you'll be in trouble. You may be tempted to search around for a suitable home medicine cure – or to see your doctor and ask for sleeping pills. Before you think about remedies I suggest that you look at the possible causes of your sleeplessness.

What's keeping you awake ?

There are nearly as many causes of sleeplessness as there are insomniacs. Very often it isn't a cure for the sleeplessness itself that is needed as much as a cure for the cause.

For example, someone who is kept awake by pain needs a painkiller not a hypnotic drug. Better than that he needs to have the cause of his pain investigated and, if possible, eradicated.

Many people lie awake because they are too hot or too cold or because there is too much noise around. Solving these problems is as likely to be within the province of a plumber or carpenter as a doctor. If there are draughts have them sealed. If the heating is unsatisfactory procure some alternative, additional source of warmth. If the bed is too warm reducing the number of bedclothes may solve the problem. If there is too much noise double glazing, wall-to-wall bookshelves or ear muffs may be the answer.

Too much food may cause sleeplessness as may an overdose of caffeine, contained perhaps in a bedtime drink of coffee. Changing suppertime habits can solve that problem. If you have to get up at night to empty an overfull bladder, reducing your input of fluids during the evening can solve the problem permanently.

Tension and worry are extremely common causes of sleeplessness. The man who lies awake thinking about the papers on his desk at work or the woman who can't forget the day's problems will both lose sleep. The answer for them doesn't involve sleeping tablets as much as learning how to relax. There isn't a glib answer to that problem, but readers who seriously feel that they would like to learn how to relax might benefit from reading the chapters on relaxation in my book *Stress Control*.

Many people who take naps in the afternoon, who lie in late in the mornings and who go to bed early in the evening complain that they can't sleep. That is hardly surprising. We all need sleep but the man who needs six or seven hours' sleep a night isn't going to get that if he sleeps for three or four hours in the daytime. I remember seeing a patient in his eighties who complained most bitterly that he woke up at three every morning. After I had talked to him for a while he admitted that he went to bed every evening at eight-thirty. At the age of eighty, with few demands on his muscles, he only needed the amount of sleep he was getting. I suggested that he went to bed at eleven-thirty and slept through until six. He was happy enough then.

People who have installed television sets in their bedrooms and who lie in bed watching the horrors of the late night news must not be surprised if they find themselves lying awake for some time after they have switched the set off. Mentally stimulating or arousing activities of any kind are likely to produce restlessness. Physical activities such as sex are another matter altogether of course.

Stuffy bedrooms are difficult to sleep in and cigarette smoke from one member of a household may keep the rest of the family awake. Children who can't sleep for coughing may rest more peacefully if they are separated from smokers by closed doors.

Uncomfortable beds are another common cause of insomnia. It's worth remembering that you're likely to spend a third of your life in bed. Economies which mean spending that much time with a spring sticking into your back are not really worthwhile.

So, before you even think of treatment for your insomnia see if there is anything you can do to remove the cause. As ever, the old adage about prevention being better than cure is perfectly true.

Remedies

The most effective remedies for sleeplessness are not available on prescription or even from the chemist's shop.

If you have done everything you can to deal with all the potential causes of sleeplessness and you're still lying awake, here are some hints.

Try taking a walk half an hour before you go to bed. Walk for fifteen or twenty minutes and then, when you get back home, lie in a warm bath. If you are used to having a drink at night choose something soothing, filling and milky. A clinical research trial was done on medical students and it showed that they slept better when they drank *Horlicks*. If you've been doing paperwork try and relax with a light novel. As an occasional remedy a glass of alcohol may prove helpful. If you have a sleepless partner you can both help each other to a good night's rest since sex is probably the best form of activity for inducing satisfying sleep.

The home remedies which exist are useless unless you are convinced otherwise (see p.32). Herbal tranquillizers which are advertised for sleeplessness are unlikely to help you if the remedies I have outlined haven't proved effective. And special pillows and other devices have, in my view, nothing to commend them.

Pills which your doctor can prescribe will certainly send you to sleep but most people should use them as a short-term aid rather than a permanent solution. Using them permanently is rather like papering over the cracks. It isn't going to help you in the long term and, indeed, since the underlying problem may get worse it may do you harm. Pills should be used while you and your doctor together try to isolate and treat the cause.

SLIMMING PREPARATIONS

Most slimmers want to lose weight for two reasons: to look better and to be healthier. The second of these two reasons has given chemists' shops an excellent reason for stocking slimming products. There can be few pharmacies today which do not contain a shelf or two well stocked with preparations designed to help people lose weight.

In view of the fact that doctors seem to spend a large amount of time encouraging patients to diet it seems right to include here an assessment of some of the products available over the counter without a doctor's prescription.

Appetite reducers

Those slimming products which are described as appetite reducers and which are available without a prescription frequently consist of nothing more mysterious than roughage. They contain non-digestible, bulky, harmless materials that give the slimmer a feeling of fullness. Bran, for example, is filling but non-fattening and should take the edge off anyone's appetite. Bran tablets are an integral part of the *Simbix 14 Day Bran Plan*. Scott's *Diabisc* biscuits for slimming also contain bran.

Methylcellulose is another popular non-fattening filler designed to spoil the slimmer's appetite. It is available in the following products:

Bisks, Celevac, Methylcellulose Discs, Pastils 808, Slim Disks, Slim Disks for Men, Slim-Maid Tablets, 10 Day Slimmer Treatment, Test Sixty and *Trihextin G Weight Reducing Plan.* Other products which contain bulk-filling substances such as carrageenan, guar gum, gelatin and agar are *Prefil* and *Simbix.*

There is no doubt that these products can help. But they are expensive and you can probably get similar results by sticking to a high-residue diet (that is a diet which includes plenty of roughage). Apples, celery, raw carrots, salads, plenty of vegetables, coarse breakfast cereals and coarse breads are all useful. By adapting your diet the weight change can be made permanent rather than temporary.

Some products which contain 'bulking' agents also contain added vitamins and minerals. If the diet is reasonably well balanced extra vitamins are totally unnecessary.

Finally, remember that all these products are likely to have a laxative effect (see p.51).

Meal replacements
This is the largest group of slimming foods and includes such products as 'meals in a glass' which are designed to be 'nutritious, well balanced and flexible'. Many contain extra added vitamins and minerals.

Products which fall into this category include *Carnation Slender, Nutriplan, Simbix Meal-in-a-Glass, Slim Gard* and the *Unicliffe High Protein Diet.* These all need to be used together with a calorie-controlled diet.

Artificial sweeteners
There are a good many substances which taste sweet and have a low calorie value. Some of them are 6000 times as sweet as calorie rich sugar. Unfortunately, some of the sweetest substances happen to be poisonous. There are, however, a number of widely available artificial sweeteners.

Saccharin (300 times as sweet as sugar and discovered 100 years ago) is available as *Bisks Sweetener, Hermesetas Solution* and *Hermesetas Tablets, Mini-Sax, Saccharin Tablets BPC, Saxin Solution, Saxin Tablets, Sucron Mini-Lumps, Supasac, Sweetex Liquid* and *Sweetex Pellets.* Saccharin does have a rather bitter taste and for those who find this unacceptable there are products such as *Sucron* which contain a mixture of saccharin and sugar. The calorie saving is not as great but acceptability may be higher. In addition, low-calorie drinks (such as those described as containing one calorie a can) are usually sweetened with saccharin.

The value of artificial sweeteners can be judged from the fact that by cutting 100 g of sugar out of a daily diet 400 calories can be saved. A heavy tea drinker can therefore save 3500 calories a week (equivalent to one pound of fat a week) simply by replacing sugar in tea by a sweetener.

There are regular scares about the safety of sweeteners. Cyclamates, for example, have now been taken off the market. There have been reports that saccharin can cause cancer in rats but to date there is no evidence that it can cause cancer in humans. Saccharin has been used so widely and studied so carefully that it seems unlikely that any new and particularly threatening evidence is likely to appear in the future.

Low-calorie foods

Some slimming foods are in fact nothing of the sort – they are ordinary foods that are packaged for the slimmer. In this category are those slimming meals which contain the number of calories printed on the tin or packet. These foods are handy for the slimmer who hasn't the time to count her calories herself. The disadvantage with them is that by having her thinking done for her the slimmer is never likely to learn to plan her diet on her own.

Many slimming breads, crispbreads and biscuits can be included in this category. Thinly-sliced loaves or crispbread biscuits do not themselves contain any magical slimming solution – they contain less calories than an ordinary slice of bread and the number of calories is precisely defined. Some of these products contain the almost inevitable extra added vitamins and minerals.

The slimming toffee

The theory behind *Ayds* (which contain liquid glucose and a variety of vitamins and minerals) is that by raising your blood sugar before a meal you won't want to eat as much as usual. The part of your brain that tells you that you are hungry will have been tricked. This method may well work as long as your stomach does not have a mind of its own.

Miscellaneous slimming aids

Herbal remedies are often described with a great deal of enthusiasm. For example, the *Celaton Slenda Herbal Food Supplement* is described as the 'new natural way to a slender youthful healthy body'. It contains extract of fucus, powdered butterbur, aloes, dried yeast, powdered mate, powdered uva ursi, powdered senna leaf, powdered juniper berries, powdered cascara, powdered gentian, powdered fucus, powdered rhubarb, powdered boldo leaves, magnesium citrate and sodium citrate. Most of these ingredients have a laxative action.

There are several products which include substances which have a diuretic or laxative action. Among these are *Obesettes* which contain among other things frangula (a purgative), cascara (a purgative) and phenolphthalein (a purgative); *Golden Health Slimmers Aid No. 36* which contains, among other things, boldo (a diuretic), dandelion root (a laxative) and broom (a diuretic); and *Potter's Boldo Aid to Slimming Tablets* which contain, among other things, boldo (a diuretic), cascara (a purgative) and dandelion root (a laxative).

It is true that a temporary weight loss may ensue but I do not recommend such products. The British Code of Advertising Practice states that diuretics or laxative slimming products are not acceptable because their effectiveness has not yet been substantiated.

Some companies sell creams and soaps which are said to wash fat out of the body. There is no truth at all in these claims. I can see no reason at all to recommend the use of kelp, cider vinegar or lecithin for slimming and I know of no scientific evidence that any of these products work although a lot of people *say* they do.

Machinery, etc.

There are a great many pieces of equipment on sale designed to help slimmers lose weight.

To begin with there are the exercising gadgets – rowing machines, exercise bars, cycling machines and devices such as *Slimmer-X* and *Bodytoner*. I don't recommend any of these items for two reasons.

Firstly, it is fairly difficult to lose weight simply by exercising. You need to do a great deal of exercise in order to lose weight and although firmer, stronger muscles may help keep layers of fat under control dieting is still the most important factor. Secondly, you don't need to buy expensive items of equipment (or even cheap ones) in order to exercise. Walking does not cost anything.

Finally, there are the electrical machines which tone up muscles while you sit watching TV. *Slendertone* and *Figuretrim* are in this category. I don't think anyone claims that these products result in actual weight loss without a diet being followed. They may help by stimulating better muscle control.

Conclusion
Don't waste your money buying slimming pills, replacement meals, meals in a glass or a biscuit, or special slimming foods. The only really effective and permanent way to lose weight is to eat wisely. Use low-calorie spreads, low-calorie drinks and artificial sweeteners, and eat a high-residue, low-calorie diet that is satisfying without being fattening. Buy a calorie list to give you an idea of which foods to avoid.

SMOKING HABIT

Why people smoke
There are many theories explaining why people start smoking. Curiosity, rebelliousness and an assertion of independence have all been given as reasons. Psychologists sometimes say that children smoke because they associate cigarettes with adulthood and social and sexual success.

Many smokers claim that tobacco helps them cope with difficult situations and that it enables them to manage their relationships with people more effectively. Psychologists confirm that to some extent by pointing out that smokers are usually searching for love, attention and support and that the appearance of independence and virility common among smokers in advertisements is, in fact, an entirely false one. Smokers are in reality sensitive people with only a thin veneer of sophistication and worldliness. Put at its simplest a packet of cigarettes gives the shy and uncertain individual an opportunity to make friends and meet people; it also gives him something to do with his hands!

Although all this is conjecture what is certain is that once having started smoking most people find it difficult to give up. Of current addicts less than 15% will manage to stop smoking permanently. For smokers cigarettes are a habit and a crutch. The cigarette enables the smoker to stay calm when he might otherwise panic. And, even more important, it prevents the unwelcome discomforts of not smoking. That surely is the key to the whole problem. Giving up smoking can be difficult. The smoker who abandons, or tries to abandon, his habit may become restless, tense, irritable, unable to concentrate and desperate for a 'fix'.

The hazards of smoking

Most smokers know, of course, that their habit is damaging their health. Most would be happy to give it up if they could. Since I find it difficult to avoid a little preaching here those who know all about the dangers of smoking can miss this section if they like. I'm including the sermon because it has been established beyond reasonable doubt that the most effective way to persuade people to stop smoking is to explain to them the hazards associated with the dreadful habit. So here goes.

Smoking is associated with lung cancer, bronchitis and all sorts of chest infection. Nicotine increases the heart rate and the blood pressure and puts a strain on the heart. Smoking is therefore responsible for many heart attacks and strokes each year.

Below the age of forty-five smokers are fifteen times more likely to have heart disease than are non-smokers. Cigarettes also have a bad effect on the stomach, both helping to produce ulcers and preventing the healing of existing ones. Arteries in the limbs are also damaged by cigarettes.

The Royal College of Surgeons in Britain has estimated that habitual smokers who smoke twenty cigarettes a day lose a minute of their lives for every minute they spend smoking. Put bluntly that means that a smoker who goes through a pack of twenty every day will live five years less than someone who doesn't smoke at all. Something like 40% of smokers can expect to die as a direct result of their addiction. And their final years are more likely to be painful and uncomfortable.

Smokers sometimes complain that they have known heavy smokers who have not had any trouble at all from their habit (smokers call it a habit, non-smokers call it an addiction). They also point out that non-smokers get lung cancer and heart disease!

This is rather like arguing that because some people have survived car crashes without injury there is no need to avoid serious car crashes. It is, I am afraid, one time when statistics have to be taken seriously.

A reassuring contradiction

Having completed the obligatory sermon I feel bound to admit that there is an opposing argument that deserves an airing. It doesn't often get heard.

The fact is that just about each one of us needs a crutch of some kind. Some people lean on cigarettes, others on alcohol, others on Valium and so on. There are people who lean on other people – causing *them* all sorts of heartaches. And all crutches are potentially dangerous. The man who condemns cigarette smoking may be an alcoholic.

I mention this because smoking cigarettes is bad enough. Smoking cigarettes and feeling guilty about it produces more stress, more heart disease and more illness than just smoking!

Giving up smoking

You can't buy the one thing you really need to give up smoking. And that is determination. If you really want to give up smoking then you'll probably manage it. If you aren't convinced, or certain, then you'll probably fail.

Having said that I have to add that there are many things that you can buy or do to help yourself give up smoking. And anything which helps is worthwhile.

Smokers with an economical mind will find that it helps to write down each day just how much money they have spent. It is astonishing to see just how much money is spent in a month and a year. By the end of a month many smokers will have frightened themselves into abstinence.

Another method is to change the brand of cigarette smoked every day. This makes life difficult and it makes smoking less pleasant. And it's easier to follow than giving up altogether. If you add to the problems by always buying from a different shop, buying only one pack at a time and buying in packs of ten, smoking will become quite a bore.

The best method that I've found for patients is the one which simply helps people govern their smoking habit bit by bit. This helps because it enables them to ease themselves out of the habit gradually instead of all at once.

To begin with, cut out smoking during working hours. Then stop smoking at mealtimes. Do not smoke while watching television. After a few days make sure that you do not smoke when doing anything else at all. Give up smoking in the car or on the bus. On a train or aeroplane book a seat in a non-smoking compartment.

A variation on this technique is to give up smoking room by room at home. One day swear to yourself that you will never smoke in the bedroom again. On the next day give up smoking in the bathroom. Go through the whole house room by room and soon you'll be reduced to standing on the doorstep smoking a furtive cigarette and trying to escape your own eagle eye. At that stage giving up is a relief.

There are, of course, many people prepared to take money off you as you give up smoking. The confectioners tell you to suck peppermints; hypnotists claim that they can help; and there are people making special anti-smoking drugs. Of all the methods which are available one of the most effective, according to the World Health Organization, is the placebo – an ordinary sugar pill which helps people by making them think it's helping them and which has no side effects of its own. Since the placebo depends on a certain amount of suggestion I doubt if you can successfully 'con' yourself into giving up smoking with a self-prescribed placebo. But it may be worth a try.

The commercial products on the market are undoubtedly helped by this universal effect. Here is a list of some. *Nicobrevin Anti-Smoking Capsules* contain menthyl valerianate, quinine, camphor and eucalyptus oil. *Formula 7 Anti-Smoking Aid* is a mouthwash containing silver nitrate and peppermint oil. *Heath and Heather's Anti-Smoking Tablets* contain lobelia, kola, quassia and magnesium trisilicate. *Lobidan* tablets contain lobeline sulphate which has a similar action to nicotine. If you believe in any one of these 'cures' then try it.

STINGS

Products in this section fall into one of two categories: preparations designed to help you avoid getting stung, and preparations which are intended to relieve the itching and swelling which follows a sting.

First, the preparations which are said to repel insects and thereby prevent any symptoms developing. Most have no effect on bees, wasps or hornets but are often a help in keeping midges and other small flies at bay. Incidentally, strong scents and bright colours attract insects – that's why women are often bothered more than men. Yellow seems a particularly popular colour among insects and those brightly coloured anoraks which are so common these days seem to bring the midges swarming.

Repellents are sometimes recommended for use on skin only and sometimes said to be suitable for use on clothing. The reason for this is that some repellents may damage plastics and synthetic fabrics. Whatever you buy, read the instructions carefully.

Effective repellent substances include diethyltoluamide, dimethyl phthalate, dibutyl phthalate, butylethylpropanediol and benzyl benzoate. These substances are available as sprays, wipes, creams, gels and sticks. The following products are among those which contain one or more of these substances and should prove effective: *Boots Insect Repellent* (gel and spray), *Insect Repel Wipes, Mijex, Samaritan Anti-midge Cream.*

More exotically there is now a device called *Anti-pic* which is a tiny transmitter that, according to the manufacturers, repels biting mosquitoes within a range of twenty feet.

The theory, which is devilishly cunning, is that since mated female mosquitoes (the type which bite humans) aren't interested in any advances from male mosquitoes they will be repelled by this transmitter since it makes a sound said to be like the sound of a male mosquito. It is expensive and it has to be kept going with batteries, and the manufacturers do not claim that it repels any other insects. That seems to me to be the greatest drawback, assuming that it actually works. Most of the creatures biting in Britain aren't mosquitoes.

Once you have been bitten there are many creams, lotions and sprays you can use to minimize the unpleasant effects. Most of them should work.

Calamine cream is an ingredient of *Calamine Cream, Calamine and*

Antazoline Cream, Calazean Cream, C & M Lotion and *Swarm*. Plain calamine is also available as *Calamine Lotion BP* and *Calamine Ointment BPC*. The calamine helps to cool the skin and I think that calamine creams and lotions are probably the best products to buy.

Antihistamine creams help by combating the allergic reaction which follows a sting. Antazoline hydrochloride is an antihistamine which is present in *Ayrtons Insect Bite Cream, Calamine and Antazoline Cream, Calamine and Antazoline Cream with Cetrimide, Calazean Cream* and *Cupal Insect Bite Cream*. Another antihistamine, mepyramine maleate, is present in *Anthical Cream, Anthisan Cream, C & M Lotion* and *Wasp-Eze*. Unfortunately, antihistamine creams commonly cause skin problems, such as dermatitis.

Other ingredients include cetrimide (an antiseptic) and benzocaine (an anaesthetic). *Lanacane* contains both types of ingredient. *TCP Liquid Antiseptic* is also advertised as being useful for soothing the pain of insect bites and stings.

Antihistamine tablets (such as the ones often prescribed for hay fever) may soothe itching and burning which is too severe to be helped by creams (see p.63).

Anyone who has ever suffered a severe shock reaction after an insect bite should consult a doctor about how to cope. Carrying a supply of antihistamine tablets or even an emergency injection may be a sensible precaution.

SUNTAN, SUNBURN AND SUNGLASSES

Getting a suntan without getting burnt
This isn't always an easy ambition to achieve.

When pink or white skin is exposed to the sun a number of cells are injured and release a histamine type of substance which produces reddening. After about twenty-four hours that redness slowly fades into a tan, as melanin cells migrate from the deeper parts of the skin to the surface. These melanin cells are intended to provide protection against further exposure. At the same time the skin is toughened and thickened to provide even more protection.

It is the ultraviolet light in the sun's rays which produces burning and tanning, and since these rays are not visible to the human eye, the visible brightness of the sun is not always an accurate guide to its effectiveness or danger for the sunlover.

Ultraviolet light comes in various sizes. Short wavelength ultra-violet light tends to produce a lot of redness but not much tanning, while long wavelength ultraviolet light does the opposite, stimulating the migration of melanin cells but doing a minimum of damage to the skin cells.

An ideal preparation, designed to provide some protection against sunburn and at the same time promote tanning, would, therefore, provide protection against short wavelength ultraviolet rays while letting the longer wavelength rays get through to the skin.

Chemicals which do this include aminobenzoates such as glyceryl aminobenzoate, benzophenones such as mexenone, and salicylates such as menthyl salicylate or salol.

Mexenone provides good protection because it is relatively difficult to remove with water (and so it stays on when you bathe or sweat). It is available as *Cream ER1, Mexenone Cream BPC* and *Uvistat*. Dioxybenzone is available as *Cyasorb UV 24,* glyceryl aminobenzoate as *Escalol 106* and *Nipa GMPA*, and oxybenzone as *Cyasorb UV 9* and *Uvinul M-40*. Other useful sunscreen agents include *Amerscreen P, Cyasorb UV 284, Escalol 506, Spectraban* and *Uvinul MS 40*. Aminobenzoic acid is avail-able as *Aminobenzoic Acid Lotion BPC* and as *Sunburn Cream*. There are many, many more. (I gave up when I'd collected the names of fifty products!) Prices vary a lot, so shop around.

All these products work but their efficiency varies. Many manu-facturers give their products a rating which tells purchasers how much protection they are getting. Obviously, sunbathers with sensitive skin need greater protection than those with darker complexions. It is important to remember that if kept in great heat, sunscreen agents may deteriorate (the heat inside a parked car can be enough).

When choosing a sunscreen agent read the label carefully before you buy. The product will probably contain one of the substances I've named and there should be some advice about how much extra pro-tection you are buying. Choose a product according to how easily you tan and burn.

In addition to these simple screening preparations, there are products designed actually to speed up the tanning process while slowing down the burning processes. *Bergasol* is a product in this category.

Tablets such as *Sylvasun* contain vitamin A (see p.180). I do not recommend these since a number of reports have shown that vitamin A tablets provide no protection against sunburn.

Dangers of the sun

Too much sunshine may seem like an impossibility to most of us, but, in fact, there are *some* disadvantages to being overexposed to the sunshine.

To begin with the sun can age human beings by affecting natural elasticity and drying the skin. (The word 'tanning' describes a process in the production of leather.) I have described the best ways to cope with dry skin on p.147.

More seriously, the sun can burn those unfortunate enough or foolish enough to spend too much time in it. Blondes are more likely to suffer than brunettes and redheads are more likely to suffer than blondes. Black people are far less likely to suffer from overexposure to the sun's rays since their skins are already rich in melanin and far less sensitive to the sun's rays.

Sunburnt skin is painful and red. There may also be swelling and blistering. It is important to get out of the sun straight away and to stay out of it. Sunburn may take several days to settle. It may help to have a cool (not cold) bath and to drink plenty of water. Blisters should not be burst. See p.96 for more details about the treatment for burns, since a sunburn is no different to any other kind of burn as far as your body is concerned.

Calamine or zinc creams (see p.160) are soothing. I don't recommend any of the special 'sunburn' creams, such as *Modantis* and *Acriflex*, many of which contain antiseptics.

Remember that to minimize the danger of being sunburnt you should accustom your body to the sun slowly. Begin with no more than fifteen minutes' exposure and build up daily.

Photosensitivity

Some people go red and burn extremely easily – after only a few minutes' exposure to the sun's rays. They are usually either allergic to sunlight or taking a prescribed drug which has caused some sensitivity.

Prescribed drugs which can have this effect include some tranquillizers, antibiotics, anti-diabetic drugs, blood pressure drugs, arthritis pills and occasionally even oral contraceptives.

The only solution, I'm afraid, is to keep out of the sun and seek a doctor's advice.

Getting an artificial tan

Before going on holiday it has become quite common for people to take the edge off their pallor by using a sunlamp, solarium or sunbed. As long as the instructions are followed to the letter, this can be a good idea. It does at least mean that no days are lost in getting the skin accustomed to the sun's rays.

The dangers usually arise when the instructions are ignored. Most doctors will be able to tell you horrifying stories about people who have fallen asleep under sunlamps and had their holidays ruined. The secret is, I think, not to rely on an electrical timer or alarm clock, but to have someone wake you up and drag you from the lamp after a few minutes.

It is also important to remember that if you are using an ultraviolet lamp regularly you are likely to dry your skin and produce lots of wrinkles. The sun ages the sunlover mercilessly.

Infrared lamps, by the way, simply provide heat – and that can be provided just as efficiently and effectively by a hot bath or hot-water bottle (see p.141).

If you can't wait for the sun and don't fancy a sunlamp, you can buy your tan in a bottle. Fake tans are really cosmetics rather than medicinal products and I have not listed the ones available here. Most contain either dihydroxyacetate or lawsone.

Sunglasses

There are, so I'm reliably told, over 2000 different types of sunglasses on the market. It is hardly surprising, therefore, that people often get confused about the type of sunglasses that are the best buy for them.

There are the polaroid ones which cut out unwanted reflections and which enable the wearer to get a much better look at the talent draping itself alongside the edge of the swimming pool. Then there are the photochromic ones which get darker as the light gets brighter and then get lighter again as the sun goes in. Mirror lenses which enable the wearer to hide behind a pair of mirrors seem to be very fashionable on the ski slopes.

There are contrasting claims for all different types of sunglasses. Some people say that you should never buy cheap ones because they will damage your eyesight; others that the lenses should be made of glass not plastic.

The truth, I'm afraid, is very simple. It just does not matter how much you spend on your sunglasses – the medical value of the cheapest can be just as good as the value of the most expensive. The more expensive sunglasses are usually more fashionable – that is all there is to it.

Naturally, it is a good idea to buy a pair that fit fairly well and comfortably. If the pair you choose don't seem to fit properly you can usually bend the arms a bit to make them either looser or tighter. Make sure that the lenses are clear and don't have scratches or defects, but unless you normally wear spectacles and want sunglasses made by your optician to your own specifications there is not much point in having special lenses. Indeed, plastic lenses probably are safer – they are less likely to break and cause damage, and remember that sunglasses are often worn during hectic summer sports.

Mirror lenses cut out a lot of light and so they are not really suitable for driving. Lenses that go dark and then go light again (photochromic lenses) are said to be a hazard because they do not lighten quickly enough when you drive into shadows or tunnels. But then you can always use the manual over-ride mechanism and take them off. Polaroid lenses cause a clash with the windscreen and some people find that distracting when driving. Don't try wearing sunglasses at night in the mistaken belief that they will cut out the glare of oncoming traffic – they will reduce your vision dangerously.

Finally, one additional word of warning: whatever sunglasses you buy and however much you pay for them don't think you can look directly at the sun. If you do that you will risk damaging your sight permanently.

SWEATING

It may sometimes be difficult to appreciate but sweating is a useful mechanism. It's the body's way of cooling itself down and increasing heat loss so as to lower body temperature. Unfortunately, there isn't time to explain all that when people on the bus start moving away from you.

And sweating isn't something you only do when you're hot. Some of the sweat glands which cover the human body (but which are gathered in greatest profusion under the arms and in the pubic area) can be triggered into action by fear or excitement.

The products available are probably better described as cosmetic than medicinal but since most of them are sold in chemists' shops I'll discuss them briefly in principle.

Antiperspirants, whether sold as sprays, creams or roll-ons, often contain aluminium or zinc salts which plug up the pores and temporarily prevent sweat escaping. Antiperspirants may cause unpleasant allergic reactions (see p.63) and irritations.

Since sweat is largely water, it is obviously not the sweat itself which smells unpleasantly. The unpleasant odours are caused by bacteria breaking down the excreted body fluids. It is impossible to remove all the bacteria from the skin without destroying the skin itself, but deodorants aim at cutting down the bacterial population. Unfortunately, the antiseptics deodorants contain may produce rashes and may themselves be inactivated by soap.

The best way to avoid the anti-social effects of sweating is to bathe daily, change clothes frequently and wear loose-fitting clothing when it is really hot.

Sweat rashes are fairly common in warm weather. They most commonly trouble overweight people since accumulations of fatty folds cause extra sweating and produce skin folds which can easily retain sweat and stay damp. These rashes may be sore, itchy, red and infected. If they get this bad then they need treatment from a doctor.

To avoid a sweat rash it's important to make sure that after bathing the skin is carefully dried. Dabbing dry is less damaging than rubbing. Sunbathing helps by drying and hardening the skin but there are obviously some areas of the body that it may not be possible to protect in this way. Ordinary baby powder can help provide some protection.

TONICS

There are an enormous number of tonics available. Some are sold as general 'pick-me-ups', advertised as being suitable for anyone feeling tired or run down. Others are prepared for more specific markets: there are, for example, tonics for the elderly, for children, for athletes, for the sexually unsuccessful and for convalescent patients. In addition, there are tonics which are designed to provide a short-term stimulus.

Traditional tonics contain bitters such as absinthium, andrographis, azadirachta, berberine sulphate, calamus, calumba, centaury, chirata, cinchona, cnicus benedictus, condurango, cusparia, denatonium benzoate, gentian, lupulus menyanthes, nux vomica, quassia, quebracho, serpentary, strychnine and strychnine hydrochloride. These substances, most of which are derived from plants, have two things in common: they give a medicine a bitter, unpleasant taste and many have no great medical worth. Some of them can be dangerous. Strychnine, for example, is commonly used as a poison.

Few of the commercially prepared tonics on sale today contain bitters although *Wigglesworth Adult Nerve Tonic* contains nux vomica, a substance which has actions identical to those of strychnine, although in the small quantities present here not dangerous. Many contain iron, vitamins, minerals and foodstuffs. Others include old-established remedies such as garlic and ginseng which have recently come back into favour. Sadly, there is little evidence to suggest that these revived therapies are any safer or more effective than less esoteric remedies.

Tonic foods

It is sometimes difficult to know when a food supplement becomes a medicine. I have chosen to include here supplementary products which are specifically said to improve health, or prevent the development of illness, since these are not usually qualities associated with ordinary foodstuffs. It is, nevertheless, important to remember that since it is perfectly true to say that the human body is composed of what is eaten health must inevitably be related fairly directly to food.

Honey, protein supplements and yeast are among the more obvious medicinal foods.

Honey is basically a mixture of sugars. Its value as a food must be considered on that basis. There is no more reason to consider it a medicinal compound than there is to consider mackerel a medicinal fish. And honey prepared by bees fed on particular flowers has no great advantage over other honeys. To say that it has is like saying that mackerel caught on the shady side of the bay are better than other mackerel.

Many of the firms selling honey are now also selling pollen as a protein-rich food supplement. You should judge its value as a food rather than for any special health-giving properties.

Sanatogen, one of the best-known tonics available, consists of casein, sodium glycerophosphate and glyceryl mono-oleate. Casein, the main ingredient, is prepared from caseinogen, the principal protein found in milk.

There are a number of other products containing proteins which are sold for convalescent patients or for people looking for a tonic. A substance called *1-7-1 Protein Powder* is sold as particularly useful for athletes. *Opothoid Protein Tablets* are recommended for use by people needing to relax and looking for a tonic. They are also said to be useful in the treatment of skin troubles, insomnia, arthritis and varicose ulcers. *Bemax* contains protein, iron and vitamins.

A recent research project carried out in America showed that athletes taking protein extract supplements do no better than athletes not taking protein extract supplements.

Yeast is used in the prevention of vitamin B deficiency. It is therefore an unnecessary supplement if your diet contains enough vitamin B (see p.180).

Yeast is of doubtful value as a tonic, and large doses may cause diarrhoea. If you really feel that it is what your body needs you can buy *Yeast Tablets BPC.*

Yeast is also an ingredient of *Bryst Brewer's Yeast Tablets, Canta-yeast, Calcium Plus, Ceeyesta, EG Vitamin Yeast, Emlab Brewer's Yeast Tablets, Hi-Lift Energy Tablets, Hi-Lift Honey and Yeast Tablets, Kaybee Brewer's*

Yeast, Marmite, Phillips Tonic Yeast, Muscleman Protein Plus Tablets, Super Brewer's Yeast, Vecon, Yeast-Plus, Yeast-Vite and *Yestamin.*

There are many other food supplements sold to help maintain health. Most of these supplements are no more useful as medicinal products than the supplements given away with the Sunday newspapers. So don't bother buying tablets or powders containing cider vinegar, kelp, lecithin, malt, molasses, rutin or safflower oil unless you particularly like the taste of them.

Lucozade can be considered a food supplement since it is a glucose-rich drink which also includes lactic acid and sodium benzoate; it is advertised as an aid to recovery so it should be mentioned. I've mentioned it.

Other health foods and special diets

If you suffer from coeliac disease, diabetes or any other disorder which necessitates a special diet, then you should seek advice from your own doctor or a hospital dietician. Some food products are available on prescription.

Patients convalescing and people wishing to put on weight may find concentrated foodstuffs like *Bengers, Carnation Build-Up, Complan* and *Wate-On* helpful. Unfortunately, it is not possible to ensure that weight is added to particular parts of the body.

Unusual eating programmes such as Zen macrobiotic diets can be dangerous, and children brought up on a limited variety of foods are at great risk of developing nutritional shortages. Generally speaking, it is more dangerous to follow a fad diet rigidly than it is to eat processed foods and their inevitable additives.

Iron

Anaemia is one of the commonest causes of persistent tiredness and a lack of dietary iron is a common cause of anaemia: two facts which provide some excuse for the vast number of tonics on the market which contain iron.

The cheapest way to take iron by mouth as a tablet is to buy *Ferrous Sulphate Tablets BP.* If the tablets are taken after food the incidence of gastrointestinal side effects is low. Ferrous sulphate is as effective as any of the other preparations available, many of which are considerably more expensive.

A large number of iron preparations include added vitamins and other minerals. Only pregnant women and patients with less common types of anaemia need to combine their iron with other products, so no combined preparations are worth buying. Iron preparations served up as exotic-looking capsules or liquids are not worth buying. Iron available as a liquid stains the teeth.

Taking iron as a dietary supplement, because your normal diet does not include enough iron, is not a sensible thing to do. It is far more sensible to adjust your diet to include enough iron in natural foodstuffs. It isn't necessary to eat spinach daily to obtain iron: if your diet includes a reasonable mixture of meat and vegetables then you'll be getting enough iron. Iron tablets, by the way, can be dangerous if taken in excess and should be kept away from children. They can kill.

One of the great dangers associated with the promotion of iron tablets is that patients can easily be tempted to treat themselves for too long. Anyone who feels lethargic, tired, weak, breathless or generally run down for more than a week or two should visit a doctor. The problem may be due to anaemia. But if it is anaemia then it is far better to let your doctor find out why you have become anaemic, to measure the level of the anaemia and to make the necessary adjustments scientifically. He may also be able to advise you on how best to avoid further attacks of the same problem. And if the symptoms are not caused by anaemia, treatment with iron may be completely inappropriate.

Many of the products which contain iron as a major ingredient are sold simply as iron preparations. Some, like *Iron Jelloids* and *Phillips Iron Tonic*, have the word 'iron' in their name. Other products like *Ayrtons IVY Tonic Tablets, Bidor Tablets, Dr Williams Pink Pills, Fernico Tonic Tablets* and *Three Flasks 'Over Forty' Tonic Tablets* also contain iron.

If you need iron tablets it's wiser, safer and probably cheaper to obtain them on prescription from your doctor than from the chemist's shop. If you think iron tablets will solve your problems and you're determined to treat yourself, then try one or two tablets of *Ferrous Sulphate BP* daily for a month. If you don't feel better by then, iron tablets aren't the answer.

Garlic

Garlic seems to have been rediscovered. It was widely used for its ill-defined therapeutic properties hundreds if not thousands of years ago, and the building of the Egyptian pyramids is said to have been done by men vitalized by garlic. It has been recommended for the treatment of asthma, arthritis, bronchitis, catarrh, constipation, leprosy, tuberculosis and whooping cough and for the banishing of worms and vampires.

More recently there has been some evidence that garlic can help cut down the amount of fat circulating in the blood and thereby help prevent heart disease.

But it is as a general tonic that garlic is usually promoted today. It is available as *Carter's Garlic Oil Capsules, Garlicels Healing Suppositories, Garlic Pearles, Garlisol, Garlisol Garlic Ointment, Garlisol Odourless Garlic Tablets, Garlodex Garlic Plus Remedy, Golden Health Garlic Oil Capsules, Heath and Heather's Garlic Capsules, Heath and Heather's Garlic Tablets, Lustys Garlic Perles, Natrodale Garlic Capsules* and *Simhealth Garlic Capsules*. There are undoubtedly other brands available.

Ginseng

Ginseng has been used for thousands of years as a tonic, restorative and panacea. There are scores of related ginseng plants and these are widely used in contemporary Chinese medicine as stimulants. In America ginseng, which is thought to be used fairly regularly by 5 to 6 million people as a tonic and aphrodisiac, is the most popular herb used without prescription for medicinal purposes. The normally recommended dose is up to 3 gm, although doses as low as 0.5 gm have been found therapeutically effective.

Rather like oenophilists ginseng advocates seem to delight in recommending specific varieties of ginseng. *Red Kooga Ginseng,* for example, is said to be grown for six years on the upper slopes of Korean mountain ranges. According to an article in the *Pharmaceutical Journal* the best ginseng used to be grown wild in Manchuria. Today, various species of this rather unprepossessing, shade-loving plant, which is related to ivy, are grown in the mountain forests of Eastern Asia, in the Eastern United States, Canada, India, Southern China and India. Normally ginseng is white or yellowish; when treated with hot water or steam it becomes reddish brown. There do not seem to be any pharmacological differences between these varieties.

During recent years a great deal of experimental work has been done on ginseng. It has been found to contain chemicals which can have an effect on the human body's ability to cope with stress, but the reports which have appeared have been conflicting and not conclusive. Little clinical research has been done and there is certainly no evidence I can find to recommend the use of ginseng. I have seen it said that ginseng has been shown to improve running and swimming abilities. The only research I can trace which suggests this was done with rats.

It is sometimes claimed that ginseng is perfectly safe but this is not strictly true. Ginseng has been shown to have hormonal properties and at least one case of painful, swollen breasts has been reported as being directly due to the use of ginseng. High blood pressure has also been associated with the use of the plant. It would be almost unique if any product existed which has only useful properties and we must assume that ginseng follows the usual pharmacological rules, that is it can be harmful as well as effective.

Ginseng is available in many different forms – it is sold as capsules, extracts, raw roots, teas and even cigarettes and injections. It is frequently mixed with vitamins, minerals, pollen and any other fashionable substances. One company sells it mixed up with 7.99% sea horse, 10.03% tiger genitalis, 9.56% doe genitalis and 12.69% deer's antler. If you fancy that mixture the product is called *Keitafo Banlon*.

Other products available include *Eletheron Ginseng, Heathrite Ginseng, Panax Ginseng, Phrodisine, Power Ginseng Capsules, Red Kooga* and *Reform Ginseng*.

Whatever the value of ginseng may be it can hardly be helped by the claims of manufacturers and retailers which sometimes become farcical. Promoters claim that ginseng is a stimulant, a sedative, and that it improves appetite, boosts working capacity, prevents cancer, helps sportsmen run faster, protects the body against radiation damage, improves sexual performance, treats diabetes, high blood pressure and nervous disorder, and enables bees to produce $39\frac{1}{2}\%$ more honey. Claims like these only arouse my scepticism.

Ginseng may well have a value as a tonic. I don't know. Incidentally, I do admit the exceptional honesty of the Panax Ginseng Company, which in at least one advertising leaflet refuses to make any specific claims for the efficiency of ginseng on the grounds that 'the pharmacological value of ginseng, if any, has not been subject to sufficient research to either substantiate or deny possible values'.

Herbal products

There are so many herbal tonics and general remedies available that a complete list would take up a completely disproportionate amount of space in this book. Many herbal remedies contain a large number of different constituents which makes it difficult to assess the value of the whole product. But whatever their medicinal value many herbal products do have delightful names. There are such compounds as *Eldermint Life Drops, Father Pierre's Monastery Herbs, Glentona Herbal Blood Purifier, Golden Health Blood Purifying Tablets* and my favourite, *Barker's Liquid of Life Tablets*.

Many herbal remedies are designed to soothe nervousness. Within this category are such products as *Becalmn, Golden Health Nerve Tablets, Heath and Heather's Mixture for Nervous Debility, Heath and Heather's Nerve Tablets, Heath and Heather's Tonic and Nerve Restorative, Natex 9 For Nerves, Quiet Life* and *Sleep Compleat*.

There are some herbal remedies which are designed to solve more particular problems. For example, *Athera* is said to help women cope with the 'change of life'.

Among the so-called homoeopathic remedies available as 'tonics' there are *Elasto Tablets* which are said to be good for aching legs and *Nervone* which is designed to relieve tension.

I have been unable to obtain satisfactory clinical evidence either to condemn them or to recommend them.

Vitamins and minerals

Vitamins are described at greater length on p.180 but they are included here simply because they are important constituents of many so-called tonics.

Many extremely well-known products are based largely on vitamins. *Phyllosan*, which is said to revitalize, energize and fortify and which has been promoted as particularly suitable for the over-forties, contains vitamins and iron. If you are eating properly you're wasting money by buying *Phyllosan*. Another product, *Biovital,* is said to be useful for busy housewives and others whose diet may not be properly balanced. That, too, contains vitamins and iron. *Minadex* is a vitamin and iron mixture advertised for 'building up children'. The ingredients are said to be the ones that doctors recommend and that is, of course, perfectly true. Whether doctors would recommend that a child who has no appetite, no energy and who gets tired easily should simply be given a vitamin and iron mixture without any investigations being done is another matter.

Pharmaton Capsules contain no less than twenty-one vitamins and minerals in addition to a special ginseng extract. *Stress B Vite Tablets* slowly release their vitamins as the body needs them and *Gev-e-tabs* contain vitamins and minerals designed to 'help you get as much out of life as you should'. *AD 70* contains over 100 ingredients and *Celaton CH3* which is a multivitamin preparation to which a number of extra ingredients have been added is recommended as a formula to prevent premature ageing.

Sunerven is recommended by its manufacturers for use in the treatment of nerve weakness, hysteria, brain-fag (honestly!), sleeplessness, nervous dyspepsia, headaches, neuralgia, etc. It contains vitamin B.

Other tonics which contain vitamins are *N Tonic, RVT Tonic Elixir* and *Sure Shield Vitorange Energy Tablets*. There are many other products which contain small amounts of vitamins and minerals.

Tonics which stimulate

Alcohol   Many people who would not dream of drinking alcohol regularly (and some who even claim to be teetotal) are firm believers in the efficacies of tonic wines. *Hall's Wine* contains a variety of vitamins and is not less than 24% proof spirit. *Sanatogen Tonic Wine,* available with or without added iron, contains not less than 26% proof spirit.

If you want to use alcohol as a stimulant and you think you can do so without endangering your health or your purse then do so, but be honest with yourself.

Caffeine   Caffeine is a genuine stimulant. It stimulates the central nervous system, the heart and the kidneys. It increases the blood supply to the heart and improves physical and mental powers. Many people have found that it helps give them energy when they've felt tired.

Balzac is said to have survived on vast quantities of strong black coffee, and on a more prosaic level I estimate that while writing this book I drank over a thousand cups of black coffee.

Caffeine is, of course, present in other drinks as well as coffee. It's in tea, cocoa and cola drinks too. A cup of tea usually contains between 50 and 100 mg of caffeine, a glass of cola contains about 50 mg and a mug of cocoa about 50 mg. A cup of brewed coffee contains between 100 and 150 mg and a cup of instant coffee rather less. This is more the dose needed for an effective stimulant action.

Like all effective drugs caffeine can have side effects. It can cause nausea, headaches and an upset stomach but the problems most commonly noticed are an inability to get to sleep and a need to pass urine more frequently than usual. Both these symptoms are fairly obvious results of the stimulant action of the drug. If drinks containing caffeine keep you awake avoid them for three hours before you go to bed.

It is possible to become dependent on caffeine and not infrequently tea and coffee drinkers notice that without their regular 'fix' they suffer withdrawal symptoms. Often they feel depressed, tired and lazy. Headaches may also be a problem. These symptoms will be relieved by a cup of tea, coffee or whatever else. They will disappear after a week of abstinence.

The advertising for *Pro-Plus* tablets honestly admits that each tablet contains 'about the same amount of caffeine as a cup of strong black coffee' but points out that tablets are easier to carry in your pocket. It is quite true that we can't all emulate Harpo Marx and keep coffee pots in our raincoat pockets! In fact *Pro-Plus* contain 50 mg of caffeine which is the same as *Dexcafex Stimulant Tablets* (which also contain dextrose), *Extra Energy Tablets* and *Wigglesworth Rapid Energy Release Tablets*. These products may provide useful short-term stimulation. Other tablets which contain caffeine include *Koladex Pick-me-up Tablets* and *Zanthine Tablets*. Many cold cures also contain caffeine as do some painkillers (see p.140).

Herbal baths

The advertising blurb tells you that if 'you're dead tired and just want to go home and slump into a chair', then 'a *Radox* bath will put new life into you'.

It's certainly true that if you are feeling tired a hot bath will help ease tensions and revive aching muscles. I don't see why putting anything into the water should have more than a placebo effect, although I suppose it's true that if your bath smells pleasant, looks a different colour or is bubbly you may enjoy it more.

Conclusion

There are many reasons for wanting a tonic. Unfortunately, there is no single product which can be recommended as a useful 'pick-me-up' for the person feeling weak or under the weather. Most of the products sold commercially rely upon the placebo effect for their worth (see p.32). If you still have faith in a particular branded tonic, therefore, it is probably worth your while buying it.

Preparations recommended as aphrodisiacs or aids for sportsmen must also be taken with hope. However, there are effective short-term stimulants for use by people wanting a quick 'lift' and unable to get hold of a cup of coffee or tea or a glass of cola. Tablets such as *Pro-Plus* should be effective.

One final word of warning: don't persist with a tonic if your symptoms persist. There are many reasons for such general problems as tiredness, malaise and loss of appetite. Making the precise diagnosis and ordering the right treatment needs a professional. No tonic should ever be taken regularly.

TOOTH TROUBLE

Toothache is the most obvious problem associated with the teeth. Aspirin and paracetamol tablets (see pp.134-9) are the best remedies for the pain and a visit to the dentist is wise if the pain recurs or does not go away. There are other remedies available, although since toothache often seems to occur at night or at the weekend getting hold of them might not be easy. Clove oil is an important constituent of *Boots Tooth Tincture, Kilpain Toothache Tincture, Parkinsons Toothache Tincture, Rayglo Toothache Tincture, Three Flasks Tooth-Ache Solution* and *Touch and Go Toothache Solution*. A plug of cottonwool soaked in clove oil can be inserted into the cavity of the pain-giving tooth for temporary relief. A glass of whisky will often provide considerable relief and may make sleep possible.

There are a large number of toothpastes available today, and choosing between ones which contain fluoride, strontium chloride or other substances may seem difficult. In the absence of strong clinical evidence in support of any particular brand of toothpaste, it is perhaps enough to choose a toothpaste by the same criteria as are used in the selection of other toilet articles: personal taste, price and brand loyalties are as important here as clinical claims, although the evidence suggests that toothpastes containing fluoride are worthwhile. I have not attempted to make a list of all the toothpastes which claim to offer better tooth care, nor have I listed the various tablets, mouthwashes and solutions which are said to help preserve teeth. If your dentist recommends one particular product then it may be worthwhile listening to him. In general, however, it is, I think, enough to point out that the best way to keep the teeth and gums healthy is to cut down sweet eating and brush the teeth regularly. Sugary drinks and sweets are the main reasons for the epidemic of tooth disease in young people. Personally, I would like to see restaurants reintroduce toothpicks, which are an excellent way to provide rough tooth care immediately after eating.

Infections of the gums are a common cause of bad breath or halitosis (see p.69). A dentist's advice should be sought if your gums bleed or are puffy, or if you have persistent bad breath.

There are as many products available for use by denture wearers as there are for people with their own teeth. The choice of a denture cleanser may be decided by your own dentist's recommendations or by your own tastes. There is not one obviously superior product. A number of products are available designed to help dentures fit better or stay in position (*CushionGrip, Snug* and *Super Wernets,* for example). If you need one of these products it may be worthwhile revisiting your dentist. Remember that the human mouth changes shape as the months and years go by and if your dentures do not fit properly you may need a new set.

VAGINAL DISORDERS

Recently the pharmaceutical industry has decided that women with vaginal disorders are worth exploiting as a potential market for products. Women have also been encouraged to use sprays and wipes purely prophylactically – in an attempt to protect themselves against possible infection. This is a dangerous nonsense, for there is no point at all in regularly using any medicament in an attempt to make the area sterile. There is a considerable risk of causing damage and irritation by using such products.

Many of the items on sale contain antiseptics and deodorants. *Bidex Cleaning Tissues, Bidex Spray, Elle Intimate Deodorant Spray* and *Femfresh Intimate Deodorant Spray* all contain chlorhexidine which I do not recommend for regular use since it can cause irritation. *Lanacane,* advertised as useful for stopping 'feminine itching', contains benzocaine, resorcinol and chlorothymol. I don't recommend any of these substances either for regular use in such a sensitive area as they too can cause irritation.

Any unusual or unexplained discharge, bleeding, rash or itching in or around the vagina needs expert treatment, not a home remedy.

VARICOSE VEINS

When your heart beats blood is pumped along the arteries. The blood which is pumped along arteries heading for the lungs *picks up* oxygen while the blood which is pumped towards the organs and tissues of the body *delivers* oxygen. Inside the strong, thick-walled arteries blood is under pressure, pumped with some urgency out of the heart and away towards every other nook and cranny of the body.

Once the blood has delivered its oxygen and picked up the waste products which the tissues and organs need to get rid of, it travels at a more leisurely pace and under much less pressure, being pumped along by the contractions of three muscles which surround the comparatively thin-walled veins. Valves within the veins make sure that the blood only travels in one direction.

The veins in the legs have the particularly difficult task of carrying blood up the legs. If the owner of the legs is standing upright then the blood has to be transported against the force of gravity. Clearly, therefore, someone who spends the day standing up is obviously going to put a greater than average strain on his or her leg veins – and consequently stands a high chance of developing varicose veins. Dentists and shop assistants are common sufferers for this reason.

There is another cause we know about. And that is one peculiar to women: female hormones. This perhaps explains why for every man with varicose veins there will be five women. Pregnancy is said to be an important influence and many women first develop their varicose veins when they are pregnant. Unhappily, those veins rarely go down completely at the end of the pregnancy. It's perhaps no wonder that the typical varicose vein sufferer is a woman shop assistant with several children.

Naturally, not everyone with varicose veins stands up a great deal or has had lots of children. In many people varicose veins develop for no very good reason at all. Approximately 20% of the population develop varicose veins and most of the time we just don't know why. It may be that they are just inherited – handed down in the family like heirlooms and Grandad's medals.

What we do know is that it is the veins at the back of the leg which are most likely to be affected and that the veins at the back of the left leg are more commonly affected than the ones at the back of the right leg. The swollen vein often aches, and because blood is not getting back to the heart efficiently the ankles often swell too.

When the problems are severe and there is persistent pain or swelling, perhaps accompanied by phlebitis, ulcers or skin troubles, then clearly surgical action needs to be considered. If the veins involved are small ones injections may help by artificially inducing the clotting of blood inside the small veins and therefore sealing them off. If the varicose veins are long ones then surgical removal may be necessary.

However, when the symptoms are relatively slight and not too much trouble they can be kept under control without a surgeon – simply by wearing elastic stockings.

Unfortunately, when the words 'elastic stockings' are used many people wince and pretend not to hear. Men, of course, don't fancy the idea of wearing stockings and women are reluctant to wear horrid thick stockings that they feel will detract from their appearance.

That's a pity for two reasons. Firstly, if varicose veins are left uncontrolled they are likely to get worse, and secondly, elastic stockings need not look like something Grandma threw out half a century ago. There are a number of firms making elastic stockings and tights which look more or less like ordinary stockings and tights when worn and which certainly don't offend the eyes of beholders.

Scholl are one of the best-known makers of elastic and support hosiery.

Their support hose (such as *Scholl Support Tights* and *Scholl Maternity Support Hose*) is made from man-made fibres and is recommended for use by people with very mild varicose veins.

Their elastic hosiery is made from rubber yarn and designed for more advanced varicose veins. There is another difference: whereas support hosiery is available as tights, elastic hosiery is usually available only as stockings. The *Scholl* range designed for moderate varicose veins includes *Nylastic Stockings* and *Nylastic Waistlength Stockings* (which are a compromise between stockings and tights) and for more severe problems they make *Scholl Soft Grip Elastic Stockings* which are said to be unnoticeable when worn under ordinary stockings.

In addition, there are below-the-knee stockings and coloured support socks for men. Other companies make similar ranges of products so you have quite a choice.

Elastic stockings, if strong enough to keep the veins compressed and to help return blood from the legs, can not only ease aches, reduce swelling and prevent the development of worse varicose veins but they can also reduce the risk of thrombosis, varicose ulcers and varicose eczema. It is important to remember that elastic stockings need to be worn all day if they are to help prevent the development of complications. Incidentally, doctors can prescribe some types of elastic stockings.

If you are unfortunate enough to develop a varicose ulcer or any skin trouble associated with varicose veins do not try treating it yourself. There are products like *Varicose Ulcer Ointment* for this purpose but I don't recommend them. Varicose ulcers can be a real problem and should always be treated professionally. It can take months to repair the damage caused by a day or two of improper treatment.

VITAMINS

Vitamins are said to cure diseases (from bad eyesight to arthritis), to prevent diseases (from cancer to the common cold), and to turn you into a better, fitter person (on the athletic track and in the bedroom).

Many of the claims made for vitamins are untrue. The plain truth is that if you eat sensibly you will get enough vitamins in your food. And if you don't eat sensibly then it won't be just extra vitamins that you'll need. You'll run into other problems long before your supply of vitamins gets low.

Vitamins are promoted for use by old people, sportsmen and

smokers. There are special products advertised for children ('specially combined vitamins formulated to supplement children's diets during their growing years when they can become fussy and faddy about food'), for women taking the contraceptive pill ('a balanced combination of vitamins and minerals such as zinc, specially formulated for women taking the pill'), and for slimmers (who are said to need vitamin supplements to stay healthy).

Vitamins – a short explanation

When vitamins were first discovered half a century ago they were given letters as they were identified.

So scientists produced vitamins A, B, C and D.

Then they discovered that the substance called vitamin B actually consisted of several different substances. So they began to rename the different vitamins in the B group, calling them B1, B2, B3, B4, B5, B6 and eventually getting to B12.

To everyone's embarrassment scientists later found that the vitamins they'd called B3, B5, and B7 onwards were not separate substances after all! And that is why we now have Vitamins B1, B2, B6 and B12. (There is actually a B4 as well but the rest are now simply gaps.) Just to add to the confusion vitamins in the B group are also given names. So B1 is also known as aneurine or thiamine, B2 is riboflavin, B6 is pyridoxine and B12 is cyanocobalamin.

Although there are so many different vitamins now isolated the most important ones are A, B, C and D. Some manufacturers make a great fuss of vitamins F and P. The medicinal qualities of these vitamins puts them into the same category as elbow grease!

Why you need vitamins

Vitamins are as essential to your body as oil is to your car.

Vitamin A is needed to keep your skin and eyes healthy.

Vitamin B is essential if your body is to make proper use of foodstuffs.

Vitamin C is needed for the development and maintenance of body tissues.

Vitamin D is vital to help your body turn calcium into bone.

Vitamin E is probably essential. However, we don't know why.

Getting the vitamins you need

It is not easy to become vitamin deficient.

Your body needs only minute quantities of these essential substances and many of them are available in so many different foodstuffs that experimental scientists have had great difficulty in designing diets which create a vitamin shortage in the people who follow them.

Even concentration camp inmates, desperately short of food, and underweight, have turned out to have had a satisfactory intake of vitamins.

There is vitamin A in milk, eggs, butter, cheese, liver and fish oils but if you're a vegetarian (or even a vegan – that is a vegetarian who does not even eat animal products like milk and cheese) you can get supplies of this vitamin from vegetables which contain carotene, a substance which can be converted in your body into vitamin A.

Vitamin B (which covers the several different substances known as vitamin B1, B2, B6 and B12) is found in a wide range of foods, which include both animal and vegetable products. A shortage of B1 can result in a disease known as beri-beri. You'll be safe enough if your diet includes cereals. Even refined flour has vitamins added to make up for what has been lost in the polishing.

Although beri-beri is found commonly in some parts of the world where food supplies are permanently poor it is usually only found in Britain in people who cannot absorb the vitamin because of some fault in their intestinal tract. Taking extra vitamin tablets won't help this problem at all.

Vitamin C is found in a wide variety of fruit and vegetables. Unless you never eat fresh fruit and always overcook your green vegetables you won't develop scurvy – the disease associated with vitamin C deficiency.

Vitamin D is present in cheese, butter, margarine, fish and animal livers, and oils. There is also enough sunshine even in the darkest North of England to provide most people with a good proportion of the vitamin D that they need.

A good diet

If your diet includes regular: meat, fish or eggs; fruit or vegetables; milk or cheese; margarine or butter; and cereal-based foods, then you won't run short of vitamins.

If a little makes you fit surely more will make you fitter!

This argument, that if a shortage of a vitamin makes you ill and a sufficiency makes you well then a surfeit should make you superfit, is totally illogical.

It's like suggesting that if you put 500,000 volts into the TV set you will get a better picture or that if you could pump 1000 gallons of petrol into a Mini it would go faster.

If you take more vitamins than you need you will at best be wasting your money and at worst endangering your health.

The dangers of taking extra vitamins

Vitamins B and C are soluble in water and they are therefore quickly excreted if taken in excess. Consequently overdosage isn't too dangerous. Vitamins A, D and E are, however, stored in the body and if too many supplements containing these vitamins are taken real problems can arise. Take too much vitamin A and you're likely to show the same signs as you would have exhibited had you been vitamin A deficient. Headaches, blurred vision, dry skin and hair loss can occur. Too much vitamin D can be fatal. Even a relatively low additional dosage for a fortnight can prove fatal. Children are particularly susceptible to overdosage. Multivitamin capsules and tablets may contain vitamins A and D with the result that the well-intentioned parent can easily poison an otherwise healthy child. Vitamin E in excess can cause abdominal pain, diarrhoea and lethargy.

The point cannot be made too often: anyone who is vitamin deficient needs to see a doctor to have the correct amount of vitamins prescribed and any subsequent improvement monitored precisely. If you think that you may be vitamin deficient see a doctor. Babies and infants who need vitamin supplements should be given products provided by official clinics or by a doctor.

Vitamin A

Vitamin A is available as *A Compleat, Arocin, Simhealth, Super A, Sustain A, Vitamin A Tablets* and *Yestamin Vit A*. As always, there are undoubtedly other products in this category.

Vitamin B

Vitamin B1 (aneurine or thiamine) is available as *Super B1, Sustain B1* and *Vitamin B1 Tablets*. Vitamin B2 (riboflavin) is available as *Super B2, Sustain B2* and *Vitamin B2 Tablets*. Vitamin B6 (pyridoxine) is sold under the names *Benadon* (in both 20 mg and 50 mg tablets), *Super B6, Sustain B6* and *Vitamin B6 Tablets*. Vitamin B12 (cyanocobalamin) is sold as *Cemac, Super B12, Sustain B12* and *Vitamin B12 Tablets*.

If you want to buy tablets which contain combinations of various B vitamins your choice is much wider. You can select from *B Compleat, B Natural, Boots Vitamin Yeast Tablets, Carter's Vitamin B-Complex Capsulettes, Lanes B-Complex, Quiet Life Tablets, Simhealth Vitamin B-Complex,* and a variety of *Yestamin* tablets, which contain, in addition to yeast, additional individual B vitamins. Two products, *B-Complex with Vitamin C Naturtabs* and *Stress B Vite,* also contain vitamin C.

Vitamin C

Vitamin C (ascorbic acid) is one of the most popularly marketed and swallowed vitamins. A great deal of testimony but very little evidence has been publicized in the campaign to promote the use of vitamin C to ward off colds and flu. This has been wisely described as the 'gulling of the innocent by the ignorant'. A not inaccurate statement since there is absolutely no convincing evidence to prove that taking extra vitamin C will provide any protection against infection unless you happen to be short of vitamin C before you start. Even then it is important to realize that there is widespread agreement among reputable scientists that 10–20 mg of vitamin C a day is sufficient to keep stocks up while 50–100 mg a day will saturate the tissues completely. Larger doses (and some 'experts' suggest several grams a day!) will simply result in vitamin-enriched urine being passed and may also cause diarrhoea.

As a practising family doctor I may say that if I honestly thought that there was the remotest chance that daily vitamin C would prevent the development of colds and flu I would happily prescribe the stuff for all my patients.

Vitamin C is available in several different forms, and scores of alternative products. Here are the names of some of the available brands in which vitamin C is available as a main or sole medicinal constituent: *Balanced Vitamin C Naturtabs, Blakoe-Tabs Vitamin C, Boots Effervescent Vitamin C Tablets, Boots Vitamin C Tablets, Boots Vitamin C Tablets for Children, C Compleat, C-Plus, C Sharp, Cegrovite, Delrosa Blackcurrant and Rose Hip Syrup, Delrosa Real Orange Juice and Rose Hip Syrup, Delrosa Rose Hip Syrup, Effer-C, Frooty Tablets, Healthcrafts 1 Gram Vitamin C, Healthrite Vitamin C, Hip-C, Jackson's of Devon Centurion Vitamin C Pastilles, Linus Brand Vitamin C Powder, Natural Vitamin C Honey Chews, Optrose Rose Hip Syrup, Poten-C, Sanatogen Vitamin C Tablets, Sanatogen High C, Sertin, Simhealth C Complex Tablets, Simhealth Vitamin C Tablets, Super Rose Hip Tablets, Sustain C, Videxon, Vita Glucose Tablets, Vitamin C Powders, Vitamin C Tablets, Wigglesworth Vitamin C Tablets, Yestamin Big Vit C, Yestamin Vit C.*

Vitamin D
Vitamin D is widely available in foodstuffs, and overdoses can be fatal. It is therefore perhaps not surprising that there are few, if any, over-the-counter preparations of vitamin D.

Vitamin E
This is probably the most fashionable vitamin of the moment. It is claimed that it can be used in the promotion of physical strength, the prevention of miscarriages, the slowing of the ageing process, the production of strong children, the improvement of sexual or athletic performance, the protection against pollution, and in the treatment of muscle disorders, cancer, ulcers, burns, skin ailments, sterility, lung troubles, high blood pressure, gangrene, kidney disease, rheumatic fever, heart disease, varicose veins and strokes.

There is no evidence that I know of that vitamin E does any of these things. In fact, doctors who have studied the vitamin carefully claim that anyone not receiving sufficient vitamin E in their daily diet would undoubtedly die of some other vitamin deficiency before the vitamin E deficiency became manifest. Incidentally, doctors have pointed out that it is almost impossible to design a diet which is deficient in vitamin E. It's not surprising that vitamin E is described as the vitamin in search of a disease.

Vitamin E is a main constituent of the following products: *Blakoe-Caps Wheat Germ Oil, Blakoe Vitamin E High Potency Tablets, Blakoe Vitamin E Higher Potency Tablets, Blakoe Vitamin E Highest Potency Tablets, Carter's Vitamin E Capsulettes, E Compleat, E Major, Fort E Vite, Healthrite Vitamin E, Natex Vitamin E, Natrodale Emulsified Vitamin E Capsules, Poten-E, Pure Vitamin E Oil Rollette, Simhealth Vitamin E Tablets, Super E, Super Vitamin E, Super X 200 Vitamin E Capsules, Sustain E, Vita-E Gels, Vita-E Gelucaps, Vita-E Ointment, Vita-E Succinate Tablets, Vitamin E Bath Milk, Vitamin E Chewable Tablets, Vitamin E Cream, Vitamin E Hand and Body Lotion, Vitamin E High Potency Oil, Vitamin E Oil, Vitamin E Powder, Vitamin E Skin Cream, Vitamin E Skin Soap, Vitamin E Suntan Oil, Water Solubilized Vitamin E, Wheatgerm Oil with Natural Vitamin E Complex* and *Yestamin Big Vit E*.

Vitamin F

Some authorities do not list any such thing as vitamin F but the name has been given to a mixture of unsaturated fatty acids.

Capsules of vitamin F and skin cream containing the vitamin are said, quite sincerely I'm sure, to be able to reverse the ageing process and remove wrinkles. It is also possible that warts will disappear when painted with blancmange when the moon is full. I don't believe either theory.

Vitamin F is available as *F-500 Capsules, FF Cream* and *FF-100 Naturtabs*.

Vitamin combinations

Vitamins A and D are available in combination as *Cupal Halibut Liver Oil Capsules, Healthrite Vitamins A and D, Scott's Cod Liver Oil Capsules, Scott's Emulsion, Simhealth Bone Meal Tablets, Super Cod Liver Oil* and *Super Halibut Liver Oil*.

Vitamins A, D and C are available as *Halaurant, Haliborange Tablets, Healthcrafts ADC Vits, Maws Orange Halibut Vitamins ADC, Orange and Halibut Vitamins, Sanatogen Junior Vitamins, Sunnimax, Vitamal Pellets, Vitocee Tablets* and *Wigglesworth Compound Vitamin ACD Tablets.*

Other substances in which vitamins are mixed include the following products (some of which also contain minerals): *Anduvite Multiplex Capsules, Biovital Liquid and Tablets, Blakoe Multivitamin and Mineral Diet Supplement Tablets, Blakogerm, Cantamac, Cantavite, Dermitabs, Full B with C, Gev-e-tabs, Head High Capsules, Healthrite Stress, Healthrite Ladies Formula, Maxivits, Melody Multivitamins, Minivits, Multivitamins, Natrodale Extravite Tablets, Sanatogen Multivitamins, Sanatogen Selected Multivitamins, Seven Seas Capsules, Seven Seas Orange Syrup, Super Plenamins, Vitamins C and E Combination, Virules, Vitarnin, Vitatrop, Vita-mines, Vykmin, Vykmin E, Vykmin Fortified, VM Formula* and *Vikelp.*

Minerals

Vitamin supplements are often advertised as containing extra minerals. Zinc seems to be a particularly popular mineral supplement today.

It is worth noting that zinc supplements have been highly successful in the treatment of hypogonadal dwarfs with anaemia in the Eastern Mediterranean and Middle Eastern areas. I can find no other indication for including zinc supplements in your daily diet.

Conclusion

An article in the *British Medical Journal* dated 6 January 1923 concluded: 'Under normal conditions of life an adequate supply of vitamins can be easily ensured by including in the diet a suitable amount of "protective foods" such as milk, butter, green vegetables and fruit and no advantage is to be gained by trying to obtain these substances in the form of drugs.'

That is still quite true. As I've said before, vitamin supplements are no more good for you than the supplements given away with the Sunday newspapers. Anyone who needs extra vitamins (either because of a shortage, a deficient diet or some physical abnormality) needs a doctor.

WARTS

For some reason or other warts were a common target for midwives and medicine men in the Middle Ages. There are numerous possible remedies. It is said that a wart will go away if you tie three knots in a long straight rush, make the rush into a ring and then draw it over the wart nine times before throwing it away. If that sounds too complicated you can blow on the wart nine times when the moon is full or touch each wart with a pea on the first day of a new moon, subsequently wrapping the collected peas in a cloth and throwing them away. If you don't mind who gets your warts you can rub each of them with a thread, grain of wheat or stone and then leave the thread, wheat or stone at a crossroads. The first person to pick up the object will have the warts.

If you're braver than I you can set fire to cobwebs on top of the wart, make a mole's nose bleed and let the blood drip on to the wart, or stroke the warts with a tortoiseshell cat's tail in the month of May.

If none of those remedies works there are more modern solutions to your problems. But first a word of warning: if you have what you think is a wart but it bleeds, grows or changes colour, then you must not try treating it yourself. Visit a doctor and ask him to look at it. Warty-looking growths can turn out to be malignant and if they are seen before they have a chance to grow they can be safely and completely removed.

Most of the available remedies for warts contain salicylic acid (a keratolytic – see p.51). This is an important ingredient of *Avrogel, Ayrtons Corn and Wart Paint, Compound W, Duofilm, Salactol, Verrugon* and *Wartex Ointment. Salicylic Acid Collodion BPC* is an economical way to obtain salicylic acid but the proprietary preparations may be easier to use and often include useful instructions. Branded preparations are often prescribed by doctors. *Cupal Wart Solvent* contains glacial acetic acid which can also be used for the same purpose.

These compounds all need to be applied for several weeks to the warts. They shouldn't be used for warts on the face or genitalia but can be used with success for warts on hands or feet. (Plantar warts which are also known as verrucae are simply warts which happen to be on the feet – like warts in other places they are probably caused by a virus.)

Most warts disappear by themselves in time but if yours don't seem to be going or if you can't wait or if they're in an embarrassing or tricky place, then visit your doctor. Skin specialists have a few tricks up their sleeves for getting rid of warts.

WATER RETENTION
There are numerous symptoms of water or fluid retention in the body and hundreds of causes.

Swelling of the ankles is probably the commonest symptom. It is a problem that often occurs in women who are overweight, aged between thirty and fifty and on their feet a lot in the day. By itself it means nothing at all and the swelling will often disappear if the woman diets and loses weight and wears elastic stockings to help keep the swelling under control during the dieting.

But ankle swelling can mean other things. Accompanied by breathlessness, for example, it can be a sign of heart failure and requires medical attention without too much delay. Accompanied by pain and perhaps some redness it can be a sign of a blood clot. Accompanied by swelling elsewhere it can mean kidney trouble or an allergic problem. You can see that if your ankle swelling needs treatment, the treatment needs to be prescribed by a doctor!

Swelling of the breasts, abdomen and legs often occurs just prior to a period. Water is retained and the result can be discomfort and even quite severe pain. The solution for premenstrual swelling may be hormonal, or it may involve the use of special diuretic pills designed to speed up the expulsion of fluid from the body. But a precise diagnosis is needed. The breasts can swell in other conditions. In pregnancy, for example, breast swelling and fullness is extremely common. Again you should not try treating yourself with diuretic tablets.

I am all in favour of home medicines, but I can think of nothing for which I would recommend products like *Aqua Ban* or *Heath and Heather's Diuretic Tablets*.

WORMS AND WORSE
Most people seem to find the following disorders embarrassing. The truth is that none of these organisms has any respect for the economic or social status of potential hosts.

Lice

Don't underestimate lice. They helped spread typhus during both world wars and thereby managed to kill several million people. Today, head lice, body lice and pubic crab lice seem as well established as ever and outbreaks occur from time to time in the most select of establishments. Fortunately, not all lice carry typhus or trench fever and usually the main symptom is itching. Eggs can sometimes be seen but more usually the diagnosis is made after a 'scare' at a local school.

Possible treatments for head lice include *Dicophane Application BPC* and *Gamma Benzene Hexachloride Application BPC*. About 15 ml of either application can be used in a single dose to treat the normal-sized scalp, although the hair should not be washed for twenty-four hours after applying the treatment. Both products are available in *Esoderm Lotion* and *Esoderm Shampoo,* while gamma benzene hexachloride is also available in *Derbac Soap, Lorexane, Quellada Application* and *Quellada Lotion.* There are other useful treatments. Malathion is available as *Derbac Liquid, Malathion Scalp Application BNF, Prioderm Lotion* and *Prioderm Shampoo.* Carbaryl is an ingredient of *Carylderm Lotion, Carylderm Shampoo, Derbac Shampoo* and *Suleo Shampoo. Pediclex* contains both gamma benzene hexachloride and malathion.

The treatment of body and pubic lice involves the use of the same basic chemicals. It is also important to ensure that clothes, bedding and towels are disinfected. *DDT Powder* can be used but boiling, cleaning and ironing are also helpful.

Ringworm

Classically, ringworm appears on the skin as a red ring. It can occur just about anywhere on the head or body and the ring formation is caused by the healing of the central part of the infection.

However, ringworm is far more commonly found on the feet (where it is known as foot rot or athlete's foot) and in the crotch (where it is tastefully known as jock itch). The reason is that ringworm is a fungal infection and just like mushrooms these fungi like growing on moist, warm areas.

When it is the feet or the crotch which are affected the condition looks more like a bad sweat rash and the skin is peeling and discoloured. Itching is a common symptom.

To avoid the development of ringworm in these areas it helps to make sure that the skin is dried well. A plain talcum powder can help. Minor infections of ringworm confined to feet or crotch can be treated with *Balto Athlete's Foot Lotion, Canesten Cream, Canesten Spray, Mycil Ointment, Mycil Powder, Mycota Cream, Mycota Powder, Mycota Spray, Phytocil Cream, Phytocil Powder, Phytodermine, Quinoped, Scholl Athlete's Foot Powder, Scholl S1 Athlete's Foot Liquid, Tinaderm Cream, Tinaderm Powder, Tinaderm Solution, Tineafax Ointment* and *Tineafax Powder*. All these products contain ingredients which should help eradicate ringworm. More persistent or severe infections will need treatment from a doctor.

Scabies

Scabies is very common today. Itching is the main problem, usually worse at night, and it can affect just about any part of the body. It is only transmitted by close body contact and you're unlikely to get scabies just by sitting next to an infected person on a bus. Much more intimate contact is usually required. You may be able to see small burrows in the areas where itching is worst.

Benzyl benzoate is the usual treatment and it can be obtained as *Benzyl Benzoate Application BP*. This has to be painted on to the entire body and then left there for twenty-four hours. A second painting should be given a day or so later. Everyone who has been in close contact with the infected person needs to be treated.

Other useful products include *Eurax* and *Tetmosol*.

Worms

Threadworms, which look like tiny strands of white thread in the stools of an infected person, are the commonest worms in Britain and the ones most amenable to home treatment. They usually cause itching around the anus which is worst at night. To prevent their spread, it helps to wash hands frequently, to keep fingernails short and to avoid sharing towels or bedding or clothes with an infected person.

Piperazine is commonly used in the treatment of these worms. It is present in *Antepar, Cupal Worm Elixir, De Witt's Worm Syrup, Ectodyne Worm Syrup* and *Pripsen* which also contains a small amount of laxative.

It is usually suggested that two treatments, at intervals of fourteen days, are given.

APPENDIX

HOME MEDICINE CHEST

Keep all your home medicines in the same place. Ideally the cupboard should be kept locked, but if that isn't possible, then keep it out of the reach of younger children. Older children should be taught about the hazards associated with medicines.

The precise constitution of your home medicine chest will obviously depend to some extent upon your personal requirements – remember to keep special products in stock for use by children – but every chest should contain remedies in the following categories:

a painkiller (see p.134)
an indigestion remedy (see p.122)
a laxative (see p.86)
an anti-diarrhoeal medicine (see p.106)
an inhalant for catarrh and sinus troubles (see p.72)
an antihistamine cream or calamine lotion (see p.160)

The chest should also contain a measuring spoon or glass for liquid medicines, and a tin of assorted fabric plasters. Bandages (5, 7.5 and 10 cm), a thermometer, cottonwool, a triangular bandage and scissors can be added if you think you'll use them. Buy and store only small quantities of each product. If you buy 500 aspirin tablets at a time you may seem to be saving money, but unless you have a very large, sick family you're unlikely to use that many before they have to be thrown away. Discard and replace medicinal products at least once a year.

HOLIDAY MEDICINE CHEST

It may seem pessimistic to go on holiday with a bag or box full of medicines but it is worth remembering that if you take an umbrella with you when you go out it rarely rains . . .

I suggest that you include:

a painkiller (see p.134)

an indigestion remedy (see p.122) – sodium bicarbonate is useful, since
it doubles as a treatment for cystitis, while magnesium hydroxide
can also be used in the treatment of constipation

an anti-diarrhoeal medicine (see p.106) – tablets are obviously handier
than liquids

a laxative (see p.86)

an antihistamine cream (see p.160) or tablets (see p.63)

a sunscreen cream (see p.161) and sunglasses (see p.161)

travel sickness tablets (see p.144) – these usually cause drowsiness and
may help temporary insomnia

Pack all these in a small plastic container and keep them with you **not**
packed away in your luggage.

If you're going abroad, buying home medicines can be expensive
and confusing. Taking a holiday medicine chest can be particularly
useful then. Do also remember to take with you any prescribed medicines which may be required. If children are going with you take
suitable preparations for them. If you take any medicines in liquid
form then also take a measuring spoon or glass. A tin or box of sticking
plasters can be useful – particularly if you do more walking than usual
and end up with blisters and sore places.

FIRST-AID KITS

Most of the commercially prepared first-aid kits which I have seen are
quite inadequate. The ones which are sold for carrying in cars are
particularly pitiful, since the equipment they contain is unsuitable for
major emergencies.

Personally, I would suggest that before buying antiseptic creams and
finger stalls you buy and read a simple first-aid book. Once you know
the basic principles of first-aid you can do far more to help than you
can with no knowledge and a bootful of paraphernalia. Too often
roadside casualties are delivered to hospital neatly bandaged but quite
dead.

When you have acquired a first-aid book, prepare your own kit.

I suggest that it should contain a tin of assorted adhesive plasters for minor wounds (the fabric ones are better than the waterproof ones which may encourage infection by excluding air); a pair of scissors; a large triangular bandage; some safety pins; a stretch bandage and some sterilized wound dressings. A roll of medical tape (such as *Micropore*) is useful for holding dressings in place and a few tissue wipes (which do not need to be impregnated with antiseptic) are useful for cleaning around wounds when there is no running water available.

If your first-aid kit is kept in the car then it might be worth adding a few aspirin tablets and a tube of antihistamine cream. If any member of the family regularly takes prescribed pills it might also be a good idea to include a few of those in case normal supplies are forgotten or mislaid.

Do remember that aspirin tablets need to be thrown out if they smell of vinegar. They are best kept in dark, opaque bottles which keep the sun out.

MEDICAL BRACELETS AND NECKLACES

The Medic Alert Foundation was formed by an American doctor whose daughter had been given a dose of tetanus antitoxin which had almost proved fatal. To prevent anything similar happening again Dr Collins gave his daughter an engraved bracelet.

Today over 5 million people wear similar bracelets and necklaces which carry brief details of their medical condition and the telephone number of an office where more details are kept.

If your relevant medical history is short enough to be written on a small piece of paper the *Medi-Gen Information Capsule* and the *SOS Talisman* might be suitable.

These items of life-saving jewellery, suitable for diabetics, people who have allergies to drugs, and others with significant medical histories, are obtainable through many pharmacies. Family doctors should have details of the Medic Alert Foundation.

INDEX OF MEDICINES AND REMEDIES

INDEX OF SYMPTOMS